Change Management Strategies for an Effective EMR Implementation

Claire McCarthy, MA
Douglas Eastman, PhD

Contributing Editor
David E. Garets, FHIMSS

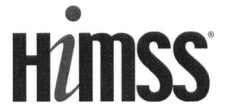

HIMSS Mission

To lead healthcare transformation through the effective use of health information technology.

Printed in the U.S.A. 5 4 3

Requests for permission to reproduce any part of this work should be sent to:

Permissions Editor
HIMSS
230 E. Ohio St., Suite 500
Chicago, IL 60611-3270
cmclean@himss.org

ISBN: 978-0-9821070-6-5

The inclusion of an organization name, product or service in this publication should not be construed as an endorsement of such organization, product or service, nor is the failure to include an organization name, product or service to be construed as disapproval.

For more information about HIMSS, please visit www.himss.org.

About the Authors

Claire McCarthy, MA, is a recognized change management/technology adoption strategist and leader with extensive experience supporting people through transitions driven by software implementations, mergers, reorganizations, process improvements, and downsizing in the healthcare industry. Ms. McCarthy works with healthcare providers and staff at all levels. She advocates for the front line, understanding that developing willingness and ability in people is what makes change successful and produces lasting results. She speaks internationally on the topic of technology adoption, encouraging healthcare leaders to invest in the people side of electronic medical record (EMR) implementations.

As Director of Organizational Effectiveness for Kaiser Permanente's national electronic medical records deployment, Ms. McCarthy introduced the concept of technology adoption to the organization and led a national community of practice focused on developing user readiness. Through integration of cross-functional work in change management, training, communication, union engagement, operations, lessons learned and workforce planning, clinical and business users were prepared to assume new roles and responsibilities in support of organizational objectives.

With 25 years of healthcare industry technology adoption experience, Ms. McCarthy has designed and led the human side of technical implementations in a wide variety of software deployments, including EMRs, practice management, material management/supply chain, client relationship management, contracting and sourcing, e-commerce, health plan product management, and, currently, ICD-10 conversion.

Ms. McCarthy is a certified William Bridges Organizational Change practitioner and is accredited in Accelerating Implementation Methodology from Implementation Management Associates, Inc. She holds a master's degree in sociology from the University of Montana and a bachelor's degree in sociology from California State University.

Doug Eastman, PhD, is an organizational development executive with extensive experience managing large-scale change initiatives. With more than 20 years of consulting experience, Dr. Eastman's focus is to help organizations grow and manage change by unleashing human potential. His specialties are organizational transformation; technology adoption and optimization; process redesign; large-scale change management; strategic planning; program and tools development; and facilitation.

As the Executive Director of Technology Adoption and Organizational Capability within the Kaiser Permanente Information Technology Care Delivery Business Information Office, Dr. Eastman currently advises senior operational and project executives on the country's largest private EMR system implementation. Dr. Eastman leverages best practices from across the program and develops implementation readiness tools and methodologies, as well as pioneering several best practice post go-live optimization strategies and programs aimed to ensure end-users are building the requisite level of system skill proficiency.

Prior to joining Kaiser Permanente, Dr. Eastman's consulting career included positions with Andersen Consulting (now Accenture), Watson Wyatt Worldwide, and a boutique employee relations consulting firm. He was also vice president of operations for a technology services firm for which he was responsible for the company's restructuring and repositioning in its marketplace that grew 200% during his tenure.

Dr. Eastman serves on the board of directors for the Childhood Anxiety Network. He holds a PhD in organizational psychology from the California School of Professional Psychology, a master's degree in psychology from Pepperdine University, and a bachelor's degree from Ohio State University.

ABOUT THE CONTRIBUTING EDITOR

David E. Garets, FHIMSS, is President and CEO of HIMSS Analytics and Executive Vice President of HIMSS. Mr. Garets has 32 years of experience in information technology. Before joining HIMSS Analytics in 2004, he was Executive Vice President at Healthlink. Prior to that, he was Group Vice President, Healthcare Industry Research and Advisory Services at Gartner. Previously, he was Senior Manager in Emerging Practices at First Consulting Group and CIO of Magic Valley Regional Medical Center in Twin Falls, Idaho. Prior to working in the healthcare industry, Mr. Garets spent 13 years in various management capacities for AT&T.

Mr. Garets was a course director and served on the faculties of the College of Healthcare Information Management Executives (CHIME) Information Management Executive Courses for 11 years. He serves on the editorial advisory boards of three healthcare information technology journals and magazines and the board of directors of HIMSS Analytics. He is an affiliate professor at the Medical College of Virginia at Virginia Commonwealth University.

Mr. Garets is a HIMSS Fellow, and was chair of the HIMSS Board for 2003-2004. He is an internationally known author and speaker on information technologies, strategies, benchmarking, and the future of healthcare. Mr. Garets has a bachelor's degree in business administration from Texas Tech University.

Contents

Foreword

By David E. Garets, FHIMSS

Electronic medical record (EMR) deployments are not about technology. They are about equipping organizations to reach critical business objectives by providing people with technical capabilities that make new things possible and by engaging people in changing their behavior to effectively use the new capabilities to generate results.

This book will show you how to create an environment for success in your organization to not only ensure that your EMR implementation effort is successful but that your organization builds change capacity and flexibility in the process. This new nimbleness will serve you well in our world of continual change.

Defining change management is as important as understanding what change management is not. It isn't project management or solely process improvement. Rather, it is a set of specific disciplines, described in detail in this book that, when coordinated and integrated, make the difference between tossing money into an EMR pit (similar to the ones that we boaters throw our money into!) or getting the sought-after changes in your organization.

Chapter 2 on Vision is especially important. In it, Claire and Doug explain how leadership paints the picture of what is expected from the implementation of an EMR. I would argue that it is a process that involves not only representatives of the front line and their managers and the senior executive team, but also the board. An EMR implementation done right—meaning the technology works, was implemented on time and within budget, and the people modify their behavior and processes to achieve commensurate value for the investment—is more transformative than anything else a healthcare organization could do. It needs to be driven from the board. That way the right people, i.e., the CEO and executive management team, are held accountable for the success of this crucial business initiative with an information technology component.

Dale Sanders, then CIO at the Northwestern Medical Faculty Foundation and now CIO at the Cayman Islands' Health Services Authority, pointed out that "you need to dedicate the time and resources to constantly iterate, refine, and improve the utilization of the EMR over time, far beyond its installation and go-live. It's a race without a finish line. Train, fund and plan accordingly—don't short-change the investment!" In other words, recognize that you are not done at go-live; you've just started achieving technology adoption and changing behavior to get value from your EMR investment.

This book should be required reading for every member of the executive team in every healthcare organization that is planning to implement an EMR in the next few years. I was happy to be asked to review the book and to write the foreword—and not for the fame and fortune! It was because I would then have to read it, and I'm glad I did. I learned an incredible amount about a topic that most of us in the technology world do not understand well and that is, dealing with people issues. Claire and Doug nail it here, and I guarantee you'll be thankful for the knowledge they share.

Having said that, reading this definitive work on change management for EMR implementations is not going to provide you with enough knowledge on the topic to preclude your engaging or hiring change management expertise. In fact, just the opposite; you'll fully understand why you need to get some help! Welcome to the epiphany.

Preface

By Claire McCarthy, MA, and Douglas Eastman, PhD

There is much discussion today about implementation of EMR systems—discussions that usually include excitement, anxiety, and downright dread. There is also a lot of talk about whether EMRs create opportunities for healthcare organizations, such as transforming the way care is delivered, reducing medical errors, increasing internal efficiencies for clinical and administrative users, improving revenue capture, and providing a host of other critical benefits. The promise (some would say fantasy) is big.

But, above all, an EMR implementation is disruptive. The process can realistically be equated to a tornado whipping through an organization, and life as you once knew it is turned upside down and the new processes, expectations, priorities, roles and methods overwhelm the workplace.

Our intent in writing this book is to assist others who may be struggling with many of the same issues we have addressed. By sharing lessons from our numerous firsthand software implementation experiences, we will equip you with successful practices and prepare you to lead or participate effectively in change management/technology adoption efforts, so that meaningful use can be achieved.

The primary audience of this book is everyone who leads or is directly involved in the people-focused change management/technology adoption efforts of an EMR implementation. Our secondary audience is everyone else who has a stake in the users' willingness and ability to change behavior so the potential of the technology can be realized. So whether you are actively engaged in change management/technology adoption work or your support and advocacy of change management/technology adoption is needed—this book is for you.

Regardless of your specific role (executive, middle-management, front-line supervisor, physician, nurse, medical assistant, IT professional, consultant, or other stakeholder in the success of an EMR implementation), our hope is that you will gain an appreciation for the importance of users and the effort required to ensure operational success. This book emphasizes effective ways to plan and implement change. The content is based on decades of combined experience managing the people side of software implementations in healthcare.

It is important to point out, however, that this book is not meant to be a course on change management/technology adoption. Our intent is not to review existing research or current academic models and theories but rather to share the insights and lessons we have learned in delivering sustainable results and healthy organizational change over the years.

For technically-oriented project leads, the success of an EMR implementation tends to focus too heavily on "screwing in the system" on time and on budget. But, as important as it is, getting the EMR technology up and running should not be the primary focus. Equal emphasis must be placed on how the new technology will be embraced, utilized, and leveraged to realize a return on this significant investment. Flipping the switch and turning the technology on is merely half of the game.

We believe the promise of an EMR implementation is great, with potentially significant returns for the patient, user, organization, and for the industry as a whole. When we hear words such as *electronic, computerized* and *automated,* it sounds as if life will be made easier and become more organized and efficient. However, healthcare organizations do not always think about the critical steps involved in making these hopes a reality. This is due in large part because managing the people side of an implementation, and developing and installing major technology require different skills sets. Neither side of the coin is necessarily more important, but they both must be seen as equally significant. The role in managing the people side of an implementation rarely fits neatly into how technically-focused projects have historically been measured, and this creates a scenario in which the people side is often misunderstood, discounted, and worst case, ignored altogether. Consider the difference between what it takes to install the system (a technology focus) and what it takes to get the desired outcomes (a focus on people doing things differently).

The management of ambiguity, resistance, and user motivation is admittedly hard to measure and unfortunately involves methods that are not always easily checked off a list. The process is more fluid and organic than linear. At times, it is unpredictable, requiring rethinking and course corrections. After all, we are dealing with people. Not everything is clear cut. Don't believe anyone who tells you it is!

People come with different backgrounds, frames of reference, experience with technology, comfort with change or ambiguity, trust in leadership, and so forth. Whatever the mix of scenarios, users never start from the same place—and they move through the change process at different speeds, meaning they continue to be in different places throughout the project. The good news is that users do grow and develop over the course of the project, and many eventually accept things they wouldn't agree to at first. But they require understanding—their fears, needs, hopes, and their reactions to the challenges that impact their ability to perform. A sound, comprehensive people strategy that creates an environment in which they can succeed is essential.

If the goal of your EMR implementation is to achieve sustainable results, growth, or organizational transformation, then a substantial investment in people must be central to your overall implementation strategy. After all, it is the user who makes or breaks your EMR implementation and ultimately determines the amount of return the organization will realize. The better prepared people are for the change and the less they see it as threatening, the faster they will deliver value.

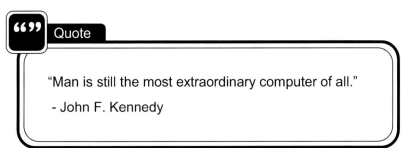

Quote

"Man is still the most extraordinary computer of all."

- John F. Kennedy

HOW THE BOOK IS STRUCTURED

Preparing an organization for a successful EMR implementation involves a big picture approach that takes into account all the factors that influence behavior change. The idea is to establish an organizational context—a culture in which desired behavior is supported and reinforced through a variety of methods—creating a learning organization that grows to achieve its vision, priorities, and goals. In this book, we present an Implementation Readiness Model and discuss each factor involved in ensuring the organization and users are fully prepared to realize the potential of the new technology.

This book is organized in a simple fashion. First, we make the business argument for change management/technology adoption, explaining why technology implementations will not deliver benefits without a significant focus on users. Next, we discuss two critical success factors in any large-scale change management effort—a clear vision and effective leadership.

Then we argue for the development of a cross-functional team of representatives from key areas within the organization, the Organizational Readiness Team (ORT), and introduce a pragmatic model that outlines the scope of complexity and work that the ORT manages throughout the project life cycle. This establishes a foundation for subsequent chapters in which each provides further detail about the inter-relationship of work involved to effectively drive sustainable change. These chapters dig deeper into lessons learned and best practices related to stakeholder management, communication, training strategy, and reinforcement, as all must be aligned to successfully satisfy the end goal of a meaningful implementation.

Finally, the Implementation Readiness chapter shows how the prior chapters serve as building blocks to formulate a comprehensive and powerful Implementation Readiness Program aimed at securing ready users who are engaged and prepared for the transitional changes ahead in the world of an EMR. The book ends with a discussion of our key lessons learned and insights regarding the overall journey. Pay particular attention to some of the larger challenges related to an EMR implementation, as these scenarios have proven to have a significant impact on an organization's speed and ability to position itself for benefits realization.

It is important to stress that focusing on just one factor of implementation readiness is not sufficient to drive organizational change and sustainable results. Each chapter describes an individual factor in detail and provides lessons and useful examples, tools, and other bits of information intended to help you succeed in preparing your organization for a successful EMR implementation. But the real purpose of the book is to raise awareness of how all factors work in concert to influence desired change associated with an EMR implementation. The factors work best as an integrated whole, overlapping and reinforcing each other. They typically have separate leadership, but whether formally integrated or not, they are pieces of one picture.

Like other books, you can jump to any chapter of interest at any point. However, we strongly encourage you to read the book cover to cover first to gain an understanding of the end-to-end process and how each factor contributes to overall success. A strategy that accounts for all factors is more effective than just one intervention or multiple disconnected interventions. In this case, the sum is definitely greater than all of its individual parts.

> **" "** **Quote**
>
> "Experience is a hard teacher because she gives the test first, the lessons afterwards."
>
> - Vernon Law

We speak to you in a conversational and straightforward manner to make this rather difficult side of an EMR implementation more approachable. We hope you will find our insights valuable and will leverage this book as your implementation reference guide. It will further your cause if all stakeholders accountable for a successful launch in your organization have a common framework for approaching the collective end goal. We certainly wish we'd had a book like this years ago to guide us through the minefield of software implementations!

Finally, we hope you enjoy the process of supporting people through the transition to the world of EMRs. There is something very rewarding about seeing people who were fearful and resistant, even in tears and thinking seriously of quitting, feel the pride of accomplishment when they succeed. Each person who stays the course and becomes a contributing member of the electronically enabled organization represents untold cost avoidance. Knowledge and talent stay in the organization, replacement costs are avoided, relationships are preserved and critical staff shortages are reduced. Technology adoption is truly a contribution to the bottom line.

In the words of one of our grandfathers, "People change when they're damned good and ready, and not before." We're here to get them ready!

Acknowledgments

The authors would like to thank the following individuals for sharing their expertise and experiences for this book:

Safaa Al-Haddad, MD
Internal Medicine
University Hospitals
Cleveland, Ohio

Ronnie D. Bower, Jr., MA
Manager, Change Management
BayCare Health System
Tampa, Florida

Nabil Chehade, MD, MSBS, CPC
Director, Medical Informatics
Regional Chief of Urology
KP HealthConnect Regional Physician Lead
Kaiser Permanente Medical Group
Cleveland, Ohio

Kenneth Goodman, MD
Associate Director, Center for Continuing Medical Education
Department of Family Medicine
Cleveland Clinic
Cleveland, Ohio

Marie Hamilton, RN
Kaiser Permanente
Oregon Federation of Nurses and Health Professionals
Healthcare Information Technology Committee, AFT Healthcare
Portland, Oregon

Lindsey P. Jarrell, FACHE
Senior Vice President & CIO
BayCare Health System
Tampa, Florida

J. Scott Joslyn
CIO
MemorialCare
Long Beach, California

Margaret M. Rudoph, PhD
Consultant
Vancouver, British Columbia
Canada

Tom Smith
CIO
NorthShore University Health System
Evanston, Illinois

CHAPTER 1

The Business Case for Change Management

"We're not in Kansas anymore…"

In the introduction, an EMR implementation is compared to a tornado in that it whips through an organization, turning life upside down and throwing users into a world filled with new ways of doing things and seeking ways to recapture some sense of balance and control. EMR technology disrupts the status quo, and along with the many opportunities it promises, it also brings a whirlwind of seemingly never-ending changes, which can have an entirely different effect on different people. While an implementation that is effectively managed even brings these challenges, a poor implementation can be disastrous and will cost the organization much more time, energy, and money to get things back on track.

Dorothy, the character from the movie *The Wizard of Oz*, held her composure pretty well through the tornado that ripped her from a calm, stable life on the farm and threw her into a foreign world. She was able to manage through the obstacles and challenges and stay the course as she followed the yellow brick road in search of the wizard. Some say this is similar to the experience users have, except for the part when Dorothy wakes up from her dream and finds herself back home as she remembers it!

EMR implementations don't have to be nightmarish for users, but there certainly will be obstacles and challenges along the way. The key is to help users through the road blocks and enable them to experience a positive journey. This process is always easier when people know what they are getting into, feel supported, and are prepared for what lies ahead, both good and bad. This is the role of change management.

CHANGE MANAGEMENT DEFINED

It's important to understand why you should make an investment in the people side of the project—bringing in the best technology possible doesn't mean anything unless users are comfortable and proficient in its use. The truth is *just because you build it doesn't mean they will come.*

Let's start by answering the two questions we are most often asked, "What is change management anyway? What is it change managers do?"

To avoid confusion we'll say up front we are not talking about change management as it relates to technical issues, such as version or change control. We also want to be clear that change management is not project management. What we are talking about is the human side of electronic medical records implementations, the human-focused work of engaging and preparing people to succeed in the new world of EMRs.

A word about project management: while good project management facilitates change management, the two disciplines are not the same. Project management is much more linear and task-focused, whereas change management deals with the complexities of human behavior. But a good project plan creates a structure and a foundation in which the change management process can occur. Therefore, the two disciplines, though different, complement and support each other.

A word of caution: do not confuse the project plan with the end result. The plan is necessary, and it guides you throughout the process. The plan is proactive; it's the order in the chaos. But technology adoption is kind of like herding cats; it's unpredictable, and you need to maintain flexibility to respond as things evolve. This is a more reactive process than what may be expressed in a plan. In our experience, an EMR implementation requires both structure and flexibility.

There is a saying in change management circles: *When one door closes another one opens, but sometimes it's hell in the hallway.* Change management deals mostly with the hallway situation, facilitating the human transition from the present to the future. These days, change is ongoing and requires focused leadership if it is to be as fast and painless as possible.

Key Tip

Our assumption is that the software you are implementing works. If the software doesn't work, you have another kind of problem—one that even the best change management won't resolve.

The three legs of the project stool represent the critical components of an implementation (Figure 1-1)—People, Process, and Technology. The people are the most important! When technology projects fail, it is primarily due to a lack of use and not a failure of the software. The focus of change management is people and the objective is to change behavior. This is good for business because it accelerates the change process so benefits are achieved faster. Change management is not about being nice or placing an emphasis on feelings. It's about performance improvement and results.

If you search the literature, you will find a variety of definitions of human-focused change management. They all cover similar concepts, sometimes using different terminology. The simplest explanation of change management is to say, "It's all about the people!" But for the purposes of this book, we expand on that concept and use the following definition of **change management:**

- A structured process designed to deal directly and intentionally with the human factors involved in not just planning and implementing an EMR but through *behavior change,* achieving the anticipated benefits that justified the project in the first place.
- Desired *behavior change* is achieved by helping people understand and internalize change and by preparing them to be successful contributors in the future state. In the case of EMR implementations, effective change management delivers users who are willing and able to use an EMR in a way that satisfies the requirements of the job, the needs of the patient, and the health of the organization.

Figure 1-1: The Three-legged Stool

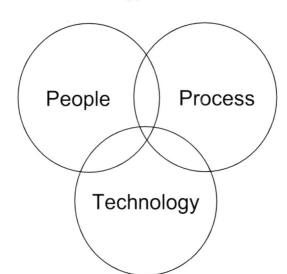

Well-designed, integrated, people-focused work builds logically over time in a way that makes sense to the user. It brings users along, guiding and supporting them so they arrive at where you want them to be. This is about willingness and ability, hearts and minds. You must have both!

The overarching purpose of change management is to **accelerate the speed at which people move successfully through the change process so that anticipated benefits are achieved faster**. And there are additional benefits to change management. Through optimizing the efficiency and efficacy of users, an effective EMR change management program will also:

- Improve organizational outcomes and performance (effective use of the system generates value to patients and the organization).
- Enhance employee satisfaction, morale, and engagement (when people learn new skills, meet performance expectations, and contribute to a greater good they feel pride in their accomplishments).
- Improve service quality (users feel valued and supported by an organization that makes an investment in them; this positively impacts how they treat patients).

- Help achieve hoped-for benefits (benefits that include EMR value realization, reduction of errors, return on investment).
- Create higher levels of openness, trust, involvement, and teamwork (develop an engaged workforce).
- Build change capability and capacity in the organization, resulting in improved ability to respond quickly and effectively to new situations (create organizational nimbleness through embedded change management knowledge, structure, and process).

In other words, it really is all about the people. Intentionally managing the cultural, behavioral, and organizational changes that need to take place to make the desired EMR future not only a reality but a sustainable reality pays off on many levels in that it also facilitates organizational transformation. Building on individual capability and organizational capacity, change management results in a change-capable culture—a huge advantage in today's competitive and fast-changing world.

Change Management, Technology Adoption—What's the Difference?

There are a number of terms that people use to refer to the work involved in managing the people side of a change effort. We think of change management as the mother ship, that is, the umbrella term that embraces all specialties within the field. Similar to the various specialties or domains of service within a healthcare system, change management professionals may choose specific areas of focus. Technology adoption, specifically information technology (IT), is one such area, and it involves the application of change management principles to the implementation of IT. **The focus of this book is technology adoption, and we will mostly use this term instead of change management throughout the rest of the book.**

Effective technology adoption professionals align themselves with the operational/business side of the organization and tailor solutions that drive behavioral change and tangible outcomes. They participate in EMR implementation projects from the beginning, driving the people side of change throughout and continuing to add value post-live as the EMR becomes part of the central nervous system of the organization.

THE IMPORTANCE OF THE PEOPLE SIDE OF AN EMR IMPLEMENTATION

There are many references in the literature to failed change efforts and IT implementations. Estimates are that only one third of these projects achieve success, which means two thirds fail to meet expectations. The good news is that failure is optional, as much has been learned about why some change efforts fail and others succeed.

Here's the issue: while the change that is going to occur is an external event—the EMR implementation, a reorganization, proposed outsourcing, a promotion, etc.—the transition from old to new that those who are impacted experience is a psychological and emotional process. It is this transition that is difficult—even when a change is self-imposed or considered positive.

In the words of William Bridges, a key thought leader in management of transitions, "It isn't the changes that do you in, it's the transition after the change that does!"[1]

For an implementation team, part of the problem encountered during transition is that change is messy: people start where they are, not where we want them to be. And when considering the personnel within a typical hospital, people can be all over the place in terms of comfort with computers, stage in life, commitment to the organization, fear of change, etc. Add to this the fact that for change to be successful three things must occur. People:

• Must let go of their current reality; have an **ending**.
• Go through a confused period **in-between** (hell in the hallway).
• Only then can have a new **beginning**.[1]

To take this a step further, while IT consultants want to install the system and make enhancements, the *users* will ultimately determine how the system is used. This use is affected by human, not technical, factors:

• Different frames of reference, backgrounds, experiences with technology.
• Organizational history and experience with other large-scale change projects.
• Levels of resistance, fear, ability to deal with ambiguity.
• Degree of alignment of "What's in it for me?" for the various stakeholder groups.

- Inefficiencies uncovered because the system creates transparency.
- Workarounds that become quickly entrenched.
- Pressure to get through the day can override doing what is right.
- User work/life balance issues coming into play from the very beginning.

All of these factors create problems for implementation teams that just want to install technology! How do you effectively address the people issues? Or is it easier to just install the technology and assume that people will learn because they have to use it? Some on the implementation team may falsely assume that users of an EMR system will snap into place over time and do what is right for the organization. This thinking is a fool's paradise.

In the foreword to this book, Dave Garets made the point that EMR deployments are not about technology but about equipping organizations to reach critical business objectives by providing employees with technical capabilities that make new things possible and by engaging them in changing their behavior to effectively use the new capabilities to generate desired results.

With all due respect to the technical side of an EMR implementation, installing the technology is only half the battle. This is not to degrade the importance of the technology. The fact that we spend a lot of money researching technology, acquiring it, configuring it, installing it, and supporting it speaks to its importance. If we weren't implementing EMRs, we wouldn't even be having a discussion about EMR-related change management!

CIO Perspective

During my master's program I took an Organization Development class that really opened my eyes to peoples' needs during large-scale change. Since the OD class I have been very interested in what makes people tick and why people react in different ways to the same environment. No matter how good of an idea a large-scale technology implementation is, we will always have early adopters, average adopters and laggards. As leaders within large organizations, we have a responsibility to plan for, and respect, all types of technology adopters. Ultimately the people who work within in our organizations want a positive human experience when they are at work.

Utilizing a change management methodology enables the implementation and leadership teams to provide a positive experience during the period of significant change. By utilizing a solid change management methodology the organization promotes team communication, a safer environment for the patient, a work environment that promotes trust and an environment where people are allowed to talk about the fear of change. All of this promotes a better human experience and a much stronger work force.

… An effective change management program has meant the difference between good go-lives and great go-lives at our 10 hospitals.

Lindsey P. Jarrell, FACHE
SVP & CIO
BayCare Health System
Clearwater, FL

But implementation of the technology is just a first, and very necessary, step—because in and of itself the technology does not generate value. The technology is necessary but not sufficient for benefit realization to occur. To create value requires people, and this is why change management is so important. Too much of a focus on technology, even in the early stages, will create issues downstream. And even with the best technology, if not used efficiently, hoped-for benefits will be tough to achieve.

CIO Perspective

I've been in healthcare IT a long time and I now realize it's all about change management. What was considered soft is now hard. We know so much more about how to install technology—it's the people part we don't know well yet, and so it's hard.

J. Scott Joslyn
CIO
MemorialCare
Long Beach, CA

Remember that change is a personal experience. It is also local and individual. And it's hard—even when it's self-imposed and positive. There are no shortcuts. People have to go through the process of change in much the same way that we move through the stages of grief.[2] It can't be avoided or skipped. You can measure twice and cut once, or you can cut now and then do costly remediation later. Either way, you can't avoid the expense or time required for real change to occur.

 Quote

"No man can think clearly when his fists are clenched."

- George Jean Nathan

SYSTEMS PERSPECTIVE

Experienced technology adoption professionals embrace a systems perspective when given the assignment to drive performance, manage perceptions, and increase the utilization of new and existing technology. A systems approach is the ability to see the big picture and address the interrelationships among the variables within the fabric of the organization and influence the combined impact these variables have on organizational effectiveness. As each variable has the power to influence the outcome of any intervention, behavior change is often not sustainable because variables tend to work against one another. Effective technology adoption strategies account for this interrelationship/interdependency and aim to bring these variables into alignment as a means for driving sustainable results.

Figure 1-2 introduces the Organizational Fabric Model, which highlights the six primary threads (or variables) that are interwoven in the fabric (or culture) of an organization. The model suggests that all six threads must work in concert to successfully shape the organizational fabric. A well-woven technology adoption plan strategically manipulates these threads to influence desired change. A poorly woven plan, in which a thread or combination of threads is not accounted for, leads to disaster or, by way of analogy, will hit a snag down the road. Depending on the flexibility and durability of this fabric, a snag can result in a huge hole that detracts from the overall strength of the intervention. The intent of the Organizational Fabric Model is to stress how important it is to understand the future state, recognize how each variable or combination of variables will come into play, and develop a sound technology adoption program that appropriately influences this set of variables to reshape the fabric or culture, so desired change can actually take place.

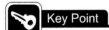

Key Point

Fundamentally, culture is "the way we do things around here."

The Organizational Fabric Model will be revisited in subsequent chapters as each thread or variable is explored in further detail. For now, we reiterate that technology adoption strategies must not rely on only one or two threads to drive behavior change. Sustainable outcomes result from an organization's ability to leverage the combination of all six threads, working in concert, to create an environment for success.

Figure 1-2: Organizational Fabric Model

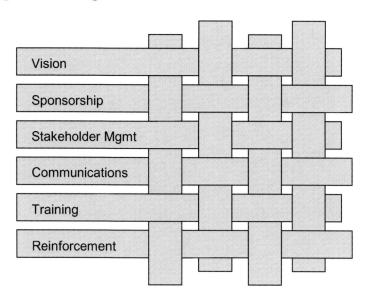

CREATING AN ENVIRONMENT FOR SUCCESS

Technology adoption is about creating a context, an environment, in which change can be achieved and sustained over the long term. This involves two levels—organizational and individual.

With an EMR implementation, the organization must create the supporting environment, provide needed training and resources, articulate a clear direction coupled with clear expectations, engage its people, include them in the process, and reinforce desired new behaviors. This is not about checking things off a list, but rather about finding synergy among impacted groups, giving them what they need, and coordinating efforts to meet the end goal. It's an ongoing effort.

To give you an idea of what we are talking about, here's an example of an individual situation occurring within a social context. Think about what happens when you want to make a significant change in your personal life—quit smoking, stop drinking, lose weight. It's one thing to talk with a doctor or another professional about what needs to happen when you're in their office, but once you leave the office you then return to your social reality. If your friends and family don't want your behavior to change, you will have a tough time. All the reinforcements and temptations will conspire to prevent you from making changes. But, if you can get some important people in your life to make the changes with you, or at least support you in the process, you have a much greater chance of success. The lesson is **don't send a changed person back into an unchanged environment if you want to see behavior change!**

Engaging individuals involves arousing two key aspects —willingness and ability. The organization must influence both in order to succeed. With the help of the Skill Versus Will Matrix (Figure 1-3), think about it this way:

- When people want to do something but don't know how, they can't (willing/unable).
- When people know how, but don't want to, they won't (able/unwilling).

Can you think of examples in your own life when you have been in either of these situations?

Consider the circumstance of people who know how to do something, but don't want to do it. This is a "will" not a "skill" issue, and it is a very common technology adoption dilemma. If the amount of work and effort involved are not perceived by the user as being equal to the

Figure 1-3: The Skill versus Will Matrix

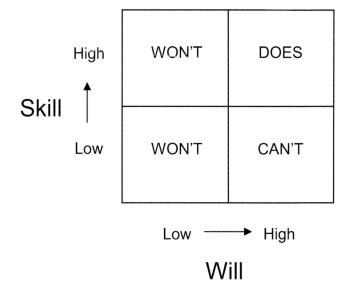

return or value experienced through the implementation, the user will most likely choose to reduce the effort. A goal of an effective people-focused strategy is to identify potential areas of disconnect and find ways to increase the perceived value to users. The assumption is that when the return is perceived to be greater, the effort increases. When there are no incentives to try harder, it may be difficult to drive desired behavior change.

The point in getting users to actively support the deployment of an EMR is about a lot more than a communication plan or feature/function training. Managing the people side of an EMR implementation requires a savvy technology adoption plan that ties sponsorship, training, communication, workflow harmonization, user support and reinforcement with the business priorities of the organization and effectively coordinates all of these activities with the user in mind—in an environment that reinforces desired behavior changes.

? Key Questions

Two key questions to remember throughout the project are

(1) How will this decision impact the user?

(2) How might it impact patients?

Consider this example:

 Key Point

> In native cultures, there tend to be rites of passage that serve to transition a person from childhood to adult status in the community. The child may actually leave the village for a day or two of contemplation, following a prescribed process. When the child returns he or she is redefined as an adult and assumes the consequent privileges and responsibilities. The entire community reinforces the person's new status; the new adult is not allowed to return to being a child whenever it's convenient, but is supported to complete the transformation to adulthood. The change to adulthood does not happen in a vacuum but is part of a carefully designed process that ensures success.

In this example, what are the key elements of this process that ensure success?

- The **picture of success,** the desired outcome, is clear—it is for the child to become a functioning adult in the community.
- How this happens is clearly defined in behavioral terms. There is a **process that is known and understood** by the entire community, including children.
- Leaders at all levels in the community agree on the **desired outcome, support the entire process,** and **actively fulfill their roles** to ensure success. Leaders include village elders and formal leaders, parents of the children, informal opinion leaders, and family members.
- The children who are about to become adults take an **active role** in their own transformation, **taking responsibility** for their success. They **receive guidance and counsel** from elders. They know and understand the transformation process and what they must do to achieve their new status. **Goals and steps are clear.** They also **understand the consequences** of not successfully transitioning to adulthood.
- If there is more than one child slated to go through transformation to adulthood at the same time they are a **peer group** and as appropriate, prepare together and support each other.

- The **entire community works together** to bring about the transformation.
- Success results in positive **reinforcement**.

The environmental context is the trump card in any implementer's hand. It takes a lot of work to create a suitable environment, but it is an essential ingredient in being able to drive and sustain change.

Willingness and Ability

Earlier we mentioned willingness and ability as key concepts in technology adoption. Willingness and ability can also be thought of as hearts and minds, or will and skill. The point is the same regardless of the terms used. People need to be supported on both an emotional level, to commit, and on an intellectual level, to be able. The question to be answered is, "What are the conditions under which users will accept and adopt the EMR?"

Let's talk about willingness first.

Willingness, or hearts, is the commitment to go forward. This is impacted by many things including the following elements:

- **Leadership:** Perceived support, or lack of support, for the change from senior executives in the company, the cascade of sponsors down through the organization, and, just as importantly, from the employee's direct supervisor.
- **Communication:** Quality and frequency of verbal and written messages that describe the desired future state: tell why the change needs to happen and what will happen if change isn't made, set clear expectations, explain how the company will prepare and support people to success, and describe local details such as timelines, etc.
- **Reinforcement:** Degree of appropriateness and timeliness of rewards for demonstrating desired new behaviors and consequences for sticking to the old ways.
- **Participation:** Degree to which users are involved, every step of the way, either directly as individuals or indirectly by being effectively represented by trusted local opinion leader peers who serve as liaisons between users and the project team.
- **Organizational History with Change:** Previous organizational experience with change—good and bad—will influence user per-

ceptions and expectations of the EMR implementation. Understanding the past is important in planning for the future.

This all sounds logical but the reaction to it can be emotional. This is where people confront their fear of failure, feeling stupid, making mistakes, etc. Remember that the change may require people to give up the very things that they believe made them successful in the past. This can be a difficult sell.

Ability, or minds, is about the actual capability to successfully meet new job expectations. This is impacted by many things including the following elements:

- **Training and Support:** In most cases, the new EMR abilities must be learned. An effective training program that is role-based and intentionally focused on preparing people to perform new job expectations is key. Just discussing desired outcomes is not enough though; we have to clearly tell people what we want them to do. This requires an intellectual understanding of *what* and *how*; a conceptual understanding is necessary but not sufficient. Most people need to practice something new to develop competence and confidence. Safe opportunities to practice, preferably with immediate feedback, are very important to proficiency development and sustainability.

Getting people to move in the direction you want is the difficulty—some say the hardest part of the whole project. And if you agree that people are the foundation of success—that benefit realization is dependant, not on technology, but on people agreeing to go through personal disruption, learn new things, change established patterns and confront their fears—then we must be proactive and courageous in addressing the human issues.

This is the people side of the project. This is the organizational readiness function. It involves collaboration, coordination and sequencing of activities, information and events from all people-focused areas. The idea is to have all the people-focused functions working together to reach clearly defined, shared outcomes. The organizational readiness plan to create individual and organizational readiness is the umbrella that connects it all—the glue that holds it together and the grease that makes it work—for the **user.** We will address the structure and process for doing this in more detail in subsequent chapters.

Good News on Two Fronts

1. There is a social science! There is a body of work, research and subsequent publications about the human experience with change. There are proven change management strategies, tools, and techniques. This isn't folklore, hooey, or black magic. The transition process is known and predictable. There is a change curve that describes the steps (Chapter 5, Stakeholder Management). And though there is no silver bullet, it isn't rocket science. Senior healthcare executives must take the emerging profession of change management/technology adoption seriously. Not understanding it is no excuse for ignoring it. That is far too expensive an option.

> "Not everything that can be counted counts, and not everything that counts can be counted."
>
> - Albert Einstein

2. All people go through transition when change—good or bad—happens, in both their personal and professional life. You can't avoid it. The wonderful thing is if you learn about change and transition at work, it will improve your personal life. This is one of the times to "try this at home!" We're all human—at work and at home. So treat your people as the humans they are, and avoid some predictable expense and difficulty. Lead your organization to a successful outcome, and speed up the process by treating your staff as customers first.

   Don't make the mistake of glossing over the critical human aspects of change. Hire experts and find the emotionally intelligent people in your organization who want to participate. And remember, you can install technology without your people, but you can't fully implement and achieve return on investment without them. **Consciously choose to move fear and resistance to trust and adoption.** It's a case of pay now or pay later. If you wait until later, it will always cost more. Technology Adoption is expensive but not as expensive as trying to gloss it over and then having to undo the damage. When failure happens, it takes a long time for people to re-engage. And in today's world, this presents real problems for healthcare organizations faced with shortages in many professions. There is a huge risk of alienating and potentially losing needed staff or in causing long delays. We can do better.

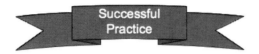

Not so long ago, it wasn't conventional wisdom that clinical application rollouts are not IT projects. More frequently than not, these were considered technical projects in which the point of celebration was when connection from workstation to central processor was reliable and wireless access actually worked. The classic IT People-Process-Technology triangle never got much past Technology to the real hard work on the People-Process axis. That has all changed in the 21st century; system implementations that are both successful and valuable have had people and process on the front burner.

When MemorialCare embarked on a five-hospital roll-out of an EMR in 2002, it had several things in its favor:

- *The technology the organization ultimately acquired was robust and reliable; it worked.*
- *It had 15 years' experience with CPOE (computerized provider order entry). Therefore, although unevenly adopted, it was not new territory.*
- *It had had the experience of a system-wide roll-out and standardization on a general finance, human resources, and materials management system. When all was said and done, users had not been sufficiently involved, standardization fell short because involvement was low, business leadership was diffuse, and IT ownership was too high. It was judged successful overall, but the organization continues to move slowly forward with an underutilized set of applications.*

With this experience and the insights of others, MemorialCare prioritized engagement of physicians, nurses, pharmacists, and other staff. Well before financial commitment to a new system was obtained, MemorialCare hired a "Care Planning Executive," a person whose full-time activities were devoted to the project, first to help understand the drivers of a new system, scope out the territory to be covered, gain the commitment of senior leaders, as well as governance, and outline the case for change. At my insistence, the Care Planning Executive, a registered nurse and former hospital chief operating officer, joined the organization, reporting to the system-wide CEO, as a peer and partner of the CIO, not a staff member, and a peer to the CEOs of each medical center campus. That dedication alone made clear the commitment, intentions, and overall priority of the company.

Among several other critical success factors—and the outcome was a success—was the overall employee engagement program that the Care Planning Executive established. In summary, it was an education, marketing, and training program dedicated to equipping the affected staff with the knowledge and tools to embrace unavoidable change. Staff communication was clear that it wasn't change for change's sake but a major move forward in the paperless way care would be delivered and workflows would be streamlined. Of course, at the time, no one could have foreseen later moves by government to push everyone in this direction (with the American Recovery and Reconstruction Act of 2009). Because of our early efforts, we're now very well positioned.

J. Scott Joslyn
CIO
MemorialCare
Long Beach, California

Leadership— Establishing a Foundation for Change

CHAPTER 2

Vision

"If you don't know where you are going, any road will take you there."
– The Cheshire Cat, Alice's Adventures in Wonderland, Lewis Carroll

Establishing and clearly communicating a compelling vision is a critical success factor in creating an effective context for change.

VISION DEFINED

The vision is the picture of the desired future state. It is the rallying point for an EMR implementation—the reason for embarking on the journey. The future state defines the overall target. It's where you're going, the context in which the implementation will take place. The more complex the change the more important it is to reach agreement on the future state—and EMR implementations are clearly complex undertakings. A clear vision motivates and helps focus decisions during the natural stresses of a large, involved project. Without a clear vision it's hard to tell where you might end up.

Common mistakes with future state vision include:

- Not developing a clear future state vision.
- Not developing the vision at the right level in the organization or conducting it as a purely senior executive small group exercise.
- Creating the vision but never cascading the message to the front line.
- Developing a vision, but not all of the organization's leadership commits to the end state.
- Not using development of the vision as a process to engage the entire organization, including patients.

- Not sharing the vision broadly and continuously.
- Failing to use the vision as a yardstick of progressive accomplishment.
- Not understanding that a vision is a creative exercise, not a financial planning process.
- Burdening the vision—too long, too much data, attached spreadsheets and the like.
- Stopping short in the visioning process—taking a technical perspective and confusing installed, functional software with the real objective (patient safety, for example).

Does any of this sound familiar?

The last bullet in the list above happens much too often in healthcare organizations. Some leaders confuse the activity of installing more software with achieving the organization's vision. The pitfall is that adding more and more technology does not necessarily help the organization get any closer to achieving the vision; it may just result in an organization that has a lot of technology. Screwing in more systems is not a guarantee the organization will work more efficiently or reach better outcomes.

Developing the Vision

In a good visioning process, leaders take the time to truly think about where the organization is heading. To help people with this, ask them to suspend disbelief for the time being, let go of current reality and think about what might be possible as opposed to what is. Some leaders have difficulty doing this because it requires stepping out of their current roles. These individuals try to operationalize every idea that surfaces to test if the idea is feasible, but this only considers a future state with current state resources and context. Don't test the ideas right away; just let them flow. Set a future state date far enough out that people don't get distracted by worrying about the short term.

A visioning session should be held off site to limit distractions and should be planned and led by people experienced in vision development. The process should be driven by the CEO and the senior executive team. The board must be involved as their engagement and commitment are required for a project of this magnitude. Other key participants include representatives from key stakeholder groups. It is important to get ideas from people up and down the organization, as well as from outside stakeholders such as patients and referring physicians. A wide variety of input will allow you to craft a vision that represents many groups. And since involvement generates engagement, people who participate feel ownership of the vision and will advocate for it within their constituencies which helps generate broad acceptance.

Remember, a good vision helps keep organizations from falling into reactive mode, provides focus and aides decision making as the project moves forward. It should serve as a guide that helps people prioritize.

Given the importance of clearly defining the future state, it's surprising how many organizations either don't do the work to develop a vision or neglect to take full advantage of a clear and compelling vision when they do develop one.

THE IMPORTANCE OF A FUTURE STATE VISION

Creating a vision is all about starting your transformational journey with the end in mind. It's a bit like planning a road trip. Knowing where you're trying to go matters just as much as knowing your starting place. These two points identify the gap that your proposed route will fill. Add the objective of your trip and you are ready to plan a route that meets your requirements.

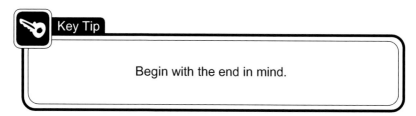

Key Tip

Begin with the end in mind.

What is your road trip objective?
- To get from point A to point B as quickly as possible?
- To do it the most fuel efficient way?
- To stop at as many museums as possible?
- To stay the fewest nights on the road?
- To hit great local food spots?
- To visit friends and family?
- To follow an historical route?

- To just have a leisurely trip and make it up as you go?

If you don't think through what you are trying to accomplish you are likely to miss the mark. The more you know about your objective the better equipped you are to plan in advance. The same is true for an electronic medical record implementation. You need a map (options), a set of objectives (vision), and roadside disaster gear (contingency plans) so you can plan your route.

The vision gives the organization a target. If you want to harness the power of your organization there is nothing like having everyone aiming at the same thing! The parts people play in the process will differ (technical, clinical, executive, etc.) but it's the vision that ties it all together.

Another advantage of having a clear vision is that it helps you plan detours when the unexpected happens. To get back to our road trip analogy, if you discover that a bridge is washed out on your carefully planned route, knowing your trip objectives will help you make a good decision about which detour to take. Having Plan B and C ready means that when something goes wrong with Plan A you won't fail because you thought through alternatives beforehand.

Take the time and make the effort to develop your vision. Do this at the beginning of the project. Use it to inspire your people, frame the project as a guide to decision making throughout the journey, and as a measure of success. Vision is the context in which the change will occur. A great vision is the glue that keeps people participating even when they'd rather throw in the towel!

VISION ALIGNMENT

These days, organizations are faced with juggling countless initiatives and priorities on a regular basis. With a clear vision, these initiatives should fall neatly into place and align with the direction of the organization. This is easier said than done, however, as it is common for organizations to try to do everything they can to increase market share or advance to the next level of transformation. The fact is that organizations cannot successfully manage and execute on everything, and must focus effort and existing bandwidth on matters that support and reinforce the desired end state.

Figure 2-1: Vision Alignment Model

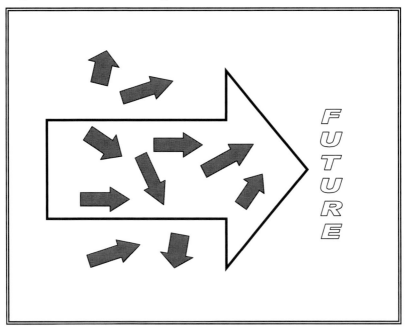

The Vision Alignment Model in Figure 2-1 reflects a view of various initiatives within the context of the bigger picture. The large white arrow represents the direction of the organization and the small gray arrows reflect the barrage of initiatives an organization is trying to manage. It is okay if each initiative is heading in slightly different directions just as long as they are inside the scope of the vision. Any gray arrow that rests outside of the larger arrow must be seen as an unwanted distraction and out of scope at the present time.

Competing priorities and initiatives that are not aligned with the organizational direction confuse and overwhelm employees. Create organizational focus by eliminating or postponing other priorities/projects to target resources and attention on the EMR implementation. Integrate related projects into the overall EMR effort. The work of prioritizing, stopping and postponing is required to focus the organization on the common goal of successfully implementing the electronic medical record system. This is a key responsibility of executive sponsors.

The completed vision must be used by the EMR project team in developing the implementation plan. This is important. Technology implementations are very involved, consisting of countless decisions, reviews and modifications. Project team members and users grow frustrated and skeptical when the project seems misaligned or haphazard. A great vision provides clear direction and helps keep everyone on track, even on bad days. The implementation plan must be tied to the vision as it is through the plan that the vision is connected to daily activities and becomes an operationalized reality.

One other suggestion: every time the vision is presented to a group is an opportunity to ask for a commitment or an action, whatever is appropriate. Think about what you most want from the group at that point in time so you are prepared to make your request. The way the group responds provides important information about their willingness to support the vision and surfaces reservations or concerns.

IT implementations are complex and involve a great deal of hard work and dedication. A clear vision helps people see the light at the end of the tunnel and makes it easier to manage through change, ambiguity, and potential confusion.

KEY ELEMENTS OF A GREAT FUTURE STATE VISION

Defining a clear vision is key for a number of reasons. The following list describes the important elements to consider.

1. Think of the vision as a picture of the future for people to step into.

To accomplish this, the vision must describe what life will be like when you reach the future state. This is a story, not a financial statement.

- How will we work?
- What will the patient experience be like?
- How will we treat each other?
- What will newspaper articles say about us?
- What will our core values be?
- Why will people want to work for our organization?
- What is our reputation?
- Why will patients choose us first?

- What will we accomplish and contribute?

It helps to use vignettes to tell stories of the future you have in mind. Make the stories personal so real people—your employees and patients—can see themselves and their families in them. If they can't relate, it won't have an impact.

2. A clear vision defines the change you are embarking on and the reasons the change is necessary.

This is where you talk about what's changing and why. Be clear about the ultimate objective of the implementation. There is a huge difference in saying that success takes place when

- The technical solution is installed and functional, versus
- Users are generating results for patients and the organization by using the EMR.

In the second definition, since user generation of results is dependant on the system, installation becomes a first step—a milestone that is required for success, but in and of itself is not the ultimate goal. After all, it's only when the system is installed and functional that the technology enabled changes can be made.

Be careful how you define success. Not doing this correctly is a key contributor to system implementation failures.

We recommend that you build your case for change, the **WHY**, into the future state vision. The case for change and the future state vision are closely connected and should not be considered separate pieces of work. Describe not only what life will be like when you reach your desired future state, but what the change is and why it must be made, why this particular version of the future was chosen, what the trade-offs were, and what will happen if you don't make the change. People also want to know who made the decision to change (e.g., the board of directors or the senior executive team), what alternatives were considered, and how the future vision links with the organizational mission. Make it easy for them to understand these important elements.

Future state is what compels people to participate. Done well it gets at both intellect and emotion. If you are going to ask people to participate in the magnitude of change required by an EMR implementation, you must answer to who, what, when, where, how, and why.

A key benefit of defining what *is* changing is that this also defines what's *not* changing. This can be a critical element for many people. Even if you are going for a full organizational transformation, building the transformation on the strengths of the current state will make the prospect less threatening for some people. Remind people what is staying the same. Honor the past and the collective journey that got you to where you are now. The future is built on your history, successes and failures, lessons learned and shared experience. All of that combines to create potential future options.

Even the most aggressive transformations are built on the foundation of the organization's history. Don't throw the baby out with the bathwater. Honoring past contributions and ways of being makes it easier to let go of them.

3. Make your vision compelling and behavioral.

We can't stress this enough. One key purpose of a vision is to engage people. This means everyone from rank and file to the most senior executives to the board. Compelling visions trigger emotions. They are not dry or technical. They make people want the future—and the best visions make people want it so much that they commit to the transformation process. If the response to your vision is, "Wow! I understand that and I want it!" your vision is doing its job!

The behavioral component is very important because it describes what it will be like in the future. This is early expectation setting and helps to draw a line of sight between where you're going and what people will be asked to do and asked to change in the process of getting there. People need to understand the connection between their performance and achievement of the vision. It is important to define the behavioral changes that will be required to make the vision a reality, and to determine the process for supporting and reinforcing the behavior changes.

In your vision sessions ask the question, "What are the most important behavioral changes we need to make for the change to be

Figure 2-2: Future State Opportunity Map

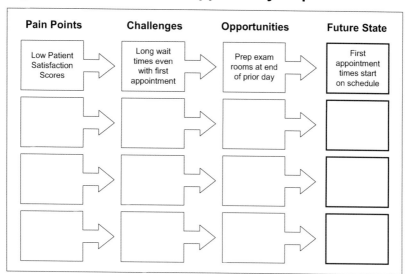

successful?" A recommended process for facilitating this discussion is to utilize a future state opportunity map.

If part of your vision is to ensure every patient experiences an excellent ambulatory office visit at your healthcare organization, based on what is known about current pain points, the group can work through identifying current challenges and opportunities for reaching a future state that supports this outcome.

Let's look at the brief example outlined in Figure 2-2. This organization is already aware that patient satisfaction scores are low from a recent patient survey. From the data, it is clear that there are several contributing factors (or challenges) that lead to an unfavorable experience for patients when coming to see their doctors. As you work with the group, try to identify opportunities and reach consensus about what the future state could look like. When individuals are involved in this future state opportunities exercise, they begin to brainstorm and find ways they can help reach the end goal. The group should explore all challenges and opportunities related to each pain point before confirming modifications to any workflows. Some challenges (when combined) can create rather complex scenarios that may need further exploration before behavioral changes can be agreed upon.

In the example provided in Figure 2-2, the team identified an opportunity to prep exam rooms at the end of the prior day as a means to ensure the first appointment of the next day can start on time. In the past, exam rooms were prepped the morning of incoming appointments, and the team found themselves struggling to get started on time. As a result, patient satisfaction scores suffered. By going through this process, the team was able to quickly see the problem, identify ways they could tweak work flows, and contribute to the vision of providing patients with a more pleasurable office visit experience. Because the team took the time to map out the scenario, they were better able to get involved and be a part of the solution.

If people understand the behavioral changes early on, and if they believe the organization is serious about improving, they may begin moving in that direction long before they are required to do so.

When the vision is compelling enough, people see the changes they need to make as worthwhile because the future is so desirable. It's amazing what people are willing to do to get something they really want! This is about more than just keeping a job, it's about working for an organization you are proud of and whose values resonate with your core.

4. Defining the end state also defines measures of success and answers the question, "How will we know when we get there?"

Another advantage of having a clear picture of the future is that you can measure against it. Use your vision to define the milestones on your journey and then report out against them as you go—use it as a yardstick. Report out even when you miss a milestone. There is no way you can get everything to happen perfectly. What you want to instill is that you are on top of it, you are paying attention, and when something doesn't go as planned you respond with a "detour" that fits with your objectives. People respect this and it builds confidence.

 Key Tip

Help people understand how you'll collectively know when you've met your target.

Give people milestones to work toward. If you are transparent about steps to milestones, individuals and departments will monitor themselves as no one will want to be seen as the reason for a miss. This is an important part of the engagement process. The vision should serve as a guide in daily decision making and prioritization, eliminating the requirement for constant supervision to ensure the right decisions are made.

Provide status updates along the way. There are few things more frustrating than working hard to contribute to something and never getting any feedback on progress. People want to feel valued and to make meaningful contributions, and they need to see that what they are doing is having an impact.

Be sure you are clear about the target you want to hit. A good way to think about this is to consider the difference between saying the goal is to get to the Super Bowl, versus saying the goal is to win the Super Bowl. In the case of an EMR implementation, the goal is not to install the system, but to leverage it to improve care or patient safety, for example.

5. **If people can't easily describe the future state to their family and friends, they don't get it.**

Finally, make your vision simple enough that it can be described in a few sentences. Distill it down by creating an "elevator speech" for people to use both inside and outside of the organization. When your employees and patients can explain what the EMR implementation is all about and where your organization is going in a way that is understood by their friends and family, they have internalized the vision. What you want is for a family member to hear about what's going on and respond by asking how they can get their healthcare from your organization.

To sum up, begin with the end in mind and communicate it in a compelling way—this is what visioning is all about.

VISION CHECKLIST

❑ Identify all the key stakeholder groups and key relationships in the EMR implementation process to determine who should have a role in vision development. Every healthcare organization has powerful constituencies. One purpose of the visioning process is to create alignment and synergy across the groups—so you must have them at the table. Engagement comes through participation.

❑ The CEO and senior executive team drives the vision process and includes the Board to ensure commitment and alignment at the top of the organization. For best results, engage experienced people to plan and lead the vision sessions.

❑ Consider using a graphic facilitator to help capture the work in pictures and make the final materials appealing. People can more easily understand and accept that they can "see."

❑ Include people from all levels of the organization in the process—and remember to include the patient perspective.

❑ This should be a collaborative process. People who participate and feel heard buy in and own the outcome. They will carry the message to their constituencies.

❑ The need and incentive to change must be greater than the desire and incentive to stay the same. You must create dissatisfaction with the way things are now without dishonoring the organization's history.

❑ Know what your organization's real passion is in making the change—is it service? Quality? Safety? Make this explicit.

❑ Be certain that the EMR implementation vision is tied to the organization's overall mission and strategic plan.

❑ Start with common agreement on what the problem is; don't jump to solutions. People don't care about the solution until they understand you care about their problem. What business and clinical problems does your EMR implementation solve?

❑ Share the vision broadly and often. Customize delivery to different audience requirements. To make this easy for people, produce a package of vision materials that include elements such as:

- Short, compelling, behavioral description of the future written in simple language. This is the "elevator speech."

- A longer document that includes more detail about the future, including stories and pictures that describe what it will be like from the perspective of patients, employees and the organization.

- A description of the process used to develop the vision and the people who participated.

- An implementation plan that will get the vision in front of the entire organization and the community to build engagement. The plan should also define how the vision will be leveraged as part of the communication strategy for the project.
❑ Remember, great future state visions:
  - Paint a picture for people to step into.
  - Are compelling and behavioral.
  - Are simple—people understand them right away without a lot of explanation.
  - Are used as a guide for decision making during the implementation.
  - Are used to define measurement of progress and final attainment of the goal.
  - Unite people around a common desire and target.
  - Define what's in and out of scope.
  - Help create dissatisfaction with the status quo while building excitement about what the organization can become.

CHAPTER 3

Sponsorship

"Be the change you want to see in the world."
– Gandhi

In this chapter, we examine the critical role effective leadership plays in ensuring the success of EMR implementations. For the purposes of this book, we refer to executives and others who are accountable for the success of EMR implementation and outcomes as *sponsors*. Sponsors use their formal authority to ensure project success.

We break sponsorship into three important levels: executive, mid-level, and front-line supervisor. We will define each level and discuss how the roles inter-relate to provide a comprehensive sponsorship network that delivers the required direction and support to the project.

Sponsorship is a critical factor in establishing context for change and ensuring a successful EMR implementation. It is not a title but a set of behaviors and actions. We are often asked, "What is the most important change management element? If we do nothing else, what do we absolutely have to have?" To which we always answer, "Effective sponsorship. If you don't have it, don't start your project."

THE SPONSOR ROLE DEFINED

Sponsorship is the single most important factor for large, disruptive organizational change efforts. Sponsors make the hard decisions, provide the budget and resources, rally the troops as needed, reinforce desired behaviors, and model the required changes.

The primary role of a sponsor at any level is to effectively communicate expectations and hold people accountable for outcomes. Here's an easy way to remember key elements of the sponsor role:

Express, Model, and Reinforce[3]

Converted to an acronym, **e**xpress, **m**odel, and **r**einforce becomes **EMR**—an easy one to remember during an electronic medical records implementation! (Pointing out this acronym [EMR] is simply an aid to help you remember the importance of these sponsorship elements *during* the implementation. All further reference to "EMR" in this chapter or within the book will refer to "electronic medical record.") Each of these three responsibilities is key to a successful project.

Express: This is what is said and includes what is emphasized, the choice of words, the level of commitment, frequency of the message, and tone of voice. Of the three (express, model, and reinforce), expressing is the least impactful. Unfortunately, it is also the easiest one to do and, consequently, the one on which most sponsors focus. The following are some important guidelines for expressing:

- Tell the truth—not your truth, but THE truth. People sense when you are not being honest about the risks and difficulties, as well as the benefits, of the pending change.
- When you don't know the answer to something, say so. Then back that up by explaining what you will do to get an answer and when you expect to provide an update.

Model: This is what you do, as in leading by example in which "actions speak louder than words." If what you say and how you behave are incongruent, people will dismiss what you tell them. Pay attention to what you do. Modeling means walking your talk. Highly effective sponsors understand the impact of making visible changes in their own behavior to model what they want to see in others. This is particularly true when the behavior change is difficult or painful for some reason. Good modeling examples include executives who:

- Publicly demonstrate collaboration and partnership in a relationship with a troubled history.
- Begin using online tools for their own healthcare transactions.
- Attend software training with staff and stay through the entire course, participating and learning along with everyone else.

- Make their incentive bonuses, and those of their direct reports, predicated on the success of the initiative.
- Admit mistakes with past change efforts and demonstrate how these learnings have informed the EMR effort.
- Openly work to improve their computer skills if they are lacking.

Modeling has twice the impact of expressing. If you are a technology adoption consultant, think about what behavior changes your executive sponsor could make that would have a big impact on your EMR implementation. What kinds of things would make a big difference at the middle leader level, and at the supervisor level? Have this conversation with your sponsors to help them see how they can increase their impact by displaying their commitment.

Reinforce: This is by far the most powerful of the three sponsor behaviors. It is also the one most often overlooked. The word *reinforcement* is carefully chosen because it includes consequences (negative) as well as rewards (positive). Yes, you must address poor performance, bad behavior, and lack of support for the project. People need to know there will be consequences if organizational expectations are not met. And as we all know, people perform better when they are acknowledged and rewarded. Reinforcement is three times more powerful than expressing. It is so important that we cover it separately in Chapter 8.

Never underestimate the degree to which words and actions communicate what sponsors value.

THE IMPORTANCE OF SPONSORSHIP

Let's start by defining what sponsorship is not. Sponsorship is not "launch and leave." We've all seen it. The executive sponsor shows up at the kick-off meeting, cuts the cake, says a few words and disappears, never to be seen again. This is not sponsorship!

When a leader takes on a sponsorship role, it is to be the ultimate owner and driver of a specific initiative. To sponsor is to be the place where the buck stops, and this can take some intestinal fortitude.

Change management methodologies often refer to leadership as sponsorship. In fact, an effective sponsor exhibits many of the same characteristics of an effective leader. The two roles overlap many ways; both have authority and credibility to:
- Be the ultimate decision maker.

- Define and enforce non-negotiables.
- Hold highest financial accountability.
- Commit resources.
- Define direction.
- Set the tone.
- Empower and hold others accountable.
- Eliminate barriers.
- Resolve the big issues.
- Provide reassurance to users.

Effective sponsorship often requires a passionate commitment to a cause. In the case of an EMR implementation, the executive sponsor is the leader of not just a software implementation but of an organizational transformation. EMRs redefine roles, ways in which clinicians practice, and the interactions and interrelationships between departments and providers—not to mention the relationships between healthcare systems; physicians and other medical providers and vendors. Patient visits and care experiences change too, as a result of the availability of up-to-the-minute patient information and the increasing participation of patients in their own care. All of these things impact the nature of the healthcare organization. Given what is at stake and what will change, we would argue that the CIO cannot be the executive sponsor, that it must be the CEO of the organization. **Note the special advice given to sponsors in Figure 3-1.**

Some question if it is really necessary for the CEO to be the executive sponsor of your EMR implementation. The answer is *yes* for three reasons:

- The disruptive and transformational nature of an EMR implementation requires leadership and direction from the very top of the organization. Actually, the very top of the organization is the board chair, but that person shouldn't have operational responsibility, other than managing the CEO!
- The amount of resources and the degree of organizational focus required for a successful EMR implementation can only be committed from the top.
- If business and clinical leaders in the organization think the EMR implementation is an IT project, they won't engage. IT is the enabler. The business must own the effort. IT provides the techni-

Figure 3-1: Note to Sponsors

Note to Sponsors

Though thinking about this can be overwhelming, it is also exhilarating because a well-designed and implemented EMR presents tremendous opportunities for a healthcare organization. We would argue that implementation of EMR systems is inevitable. So instead of worrying about whether or not to do it, put your energy into doing it in a way that provides a foundation to effectively transform your organization for 21st Century relevance. This book provides you with tools and guidelines to make you an outstanding sponsor of what might be one of the most significant professional efforts you will ever undertake.

cal foundation for transformational change, but it is the people who determine whether the effort succeeds or fails, and this is why we say that an EMR implementation is a business and clinical initiative with an IT component.

In some cases, sponsors are selected to support a particular initiative. This happens on smaller projects or when some person (or group) champions a change idea but is not in a position to become the executive sponsor. A project looking for sponsorship is very different from a large, complex, disruptive and expensive effort such as an EMR implementation. Generally, senior executives in a healthcare organization are the ones who decide to embark on the EMR journey and then authorize and initiate the project. The decision to launch an EMR implementation is top down.

If you are in a situation in which you need to find an executive sponsor for your EMR implementation because your executive leaders are not involved, you have not been working at the right level in the organization. EMR implementations cannot be authorized or initiated from anywhere but the executive suite because of tremendous expense and the degree of disruption the implementation represents. And we would further suggest that the sponsorship responsibilities cannot emanate initially from the executive suite and then get delegated off to lower echelon management. That's "launch and leave." Sponsorship must cascade throughout the organization but with senior executives retaining their executive sponsorship roles and responsibilities. Cascading sponsorship is an extension of executive sponsorship, not a replacement for it.

For an EMR implementation, sponsorship is shared among the senior executives. The CEO should remain the desk at which the buck stops and should be active in the oversight and leadership of the initiative. But the chief medical officer and chief nursing officer and chief operating officer will all have important executive sponsorship opportunities in the departments and functions they oversee. So will the CIO, but we believe it is a mistake to stick the CIO for accountability of the success of the initiative beyond the area the CIO controls, which is IT—the implementation locus. That is why the CEO has to own the initiative—the CEO is the head of the organization.

In many respects, sponsors may have more at stake in an EMR implementation than anyone else. Leadership jobs are on the line with efforts as significant as an EMR. When working with sponsors who are not yet committed to the project, begin by treating them like anyone else who needs to start at the beginning. Facilitate action by helping them through the action wave, as depicted in Figure 3-2.

Refer to the Communication chapter in which this is described (see Chapter 6). Sponsors are people too; they have fears, concerns, hopes and expectations that must be addressed if they are to become effective leaders of the project. If you discover a resistant sponsor, try to get to the bottom of the resistance by building trust, listening, and seeking to understand.

Sponsors are critical to success of the implementation process. As such, it is important to ensure they are well-equipped and comfortable in their role. Avoid the mistake of naming sponsors but not providing them with training, support, and coaching. If they are perceived as ineffective or not believable, they will be unable to motivate others and drive change. Clearly identify your sponsors and provide them with the tools and resources they need to succeed.

Figure 3-2: The Action Wave

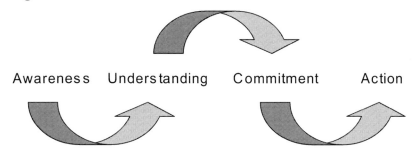

Awareness Understanding Commitment Action

SPONSORSHIP CASCADE

By breaking sponsorship into three levels (executive, mid-level and front-line supervisor), we are intentionally addressing the hierarchy of a healthcare organization. The exact terms your system uses to describe these levels don't matter, and your organization may have many more levels. What is important is that you recognize that the sponsor role is not confined to the executive suite. The role of sponsor is more or less the same at each level, but as you move up in the organization, there is an increasing span of control and authority.

To be most effective, sponsorship starts at the top of the organization and cascades down through the layers to front-line leaders. This means each successive leadership level must clearly communicate the appropriate sponsor role and expectations to the next level down. Each level must hold the one below accountable for effective sponsorship and delivery of desired outcomes.

Change efforts are always more successful when there are clear and present sponsors supporting and modeling the change. In the same way that we expect direct supervisors to provide front-line teams with a supporting, reinforcing environment in which to successfully navigate change, the supervisors themselves need the same support from their leadership to be successful and so on up the chain.

In most cases, the sponsorship cascade follows the direct reporting structure of the organization. Given this, it is surprising how often projects don't have a clear picture of their sponsorship cascade. We highly recommend taking the time to develop a sponsor map upon which you identify all sponsors of your project—up, down, and across your organization. See Chapter 5, Stakeholder Management, for information on conducting a stakeholder/sponsor mapping process.

If you miss a level in the sponsorship cascade, you will experience a breakdown in the chain. Your sponsorship chain is only as strong as its weakest link, and a break in the chain can spell disaster for an EMR implementation. It is the responsibility of the executive sponsor to ensure that sponsorship is appropriately cascaded throughout the organization. How do you do this? Highly effective executive sponsors do three things:

- Add responsibility for EMR sponsorship and outcomes to their direct reports' goals and incentive plan. This removes all ambiguity about the importance of the EMR implementation.
- Include the EMR implementation as an agenda item for each direct report one-on-one meeting and in the team meeting. The executive sponsor asks questions about the status of the project, successes, issues, staff morale, and, very importantly, how things are going for the sponsors themselves. Repeated inquiries about the activities and outcomes keeps information and accountability flowing up and down the organization.
- Manage by wandering around—informally check in with people at all levels to hear from them directly about what is working and what is not. This kind of communication and reinforcement keeps the executive sponsor close to the project, providing opportunities to assist with resource issues and problem solving as needed. It also reaffirms the importance of the project throughout the organization. If your organization has problems with "flavor of the month" reactions to change initiatives, managing by wandering around eliminates any confusion about the priority status of the EMR project.

These activities make it very clear that the executive sponsor is paying attention and actively participating. People quickly understand that the EMR implementation is a priority and that progress and status are being routinely monitored. This form of reinforcement sends loud messages across the organization.

Key Tip

Active, committed and cascaded sponsorship is critical to EMR implementation success.

LEVELS OF SPONSORSHIP

Now that we have talked about the sponsor role in general, we'll take a look at some important characteristics of each of the three levels we identified earlier—executive, mid-level, and front-line supervisor.

To begin with, all sponsors share the following responsibilities as they are appropriate to their span of control and level of authority in the organization.

Sponsor Responsibilities Shared at All Levels

- Demonstrate personal commitment to the EMR vision and the changes that must be made to get there.
- Be highly visible and consistent. Stay the course! This takes self-discipline.
- Know what results the organization is driving for and how progress and success will be measured.
- Monitor progress and ensure the project is directionally correct.
- Connect the project to the organizational strategy; draw a clear line of sight for others to see.
- Hold all players accountable for reaching desired outcomes. Make the EMR implementation a key accountability in direct report goals and incentive plans.
- Be mindful of what you communicate to peers and direct reports through what you say, how you behave, how you commit resources, what you prioritize and reward, and how you spend your time.
- Ensure open, honest, two-way communication. Engage with people to understand what's really going on. Actively listen to demonstrate that you value feedback.

- Stay engaged with direct reports to be current with project status, including successes and issues and what needs to be escalated.
- Manage direct reports' personal transition process, including managing their own resistance.
- Express, model, and reinforce the change.[3]
- Advocate for the project with peers and others.
- Actively participate in managing others' resistance and expectations about the change.
- Coach and mentor direct reports to build individual and collective capability to effectively manage today's unrelenting pace of change.
- Know how to get needed support for direct reports and their teams, and be comfortable asking for help. Understand how to make the best use of the resources available.
- Ensure direct reports understand how the change fits into their priorities. You may need to reassess and decide if some things need to come off the plate in order to create capacity for EMR success. Stop or postpone work that interferes with the EMR implementation.
- Celebrate progress and successes! Early on, look for some quick wins to build enthusiasm and confidence. Continue to celebrate accomplishments throughout the project.

Executive Sponsors

In addition to the previous list, executive sponsors have the following additional responsibilities:

- Ensure the EMR vision for the organization is clearly defined, so people understand what success looks like.
- Authorize and initiate the EMR implementation.
- Do not change priorities mid-stream. Do not shift focus, reassign resources, or create confusion. Avoid the temptation to start other initiatives before the EMR implementation is complete.
- Commit financial and human resources to the project—what gets resourced gets done.
  - For a project as complex and long term as an EMR implementation, human resource assignments must be dedicated and full-time.

– Engage an experienced change management leader to direct the people side of the project.

- Ensure effective sponsorship is cascaded throughout the organization.
- Don't underestimate what it will take to move the organization through the transition. Anticipate and help manage the resistance. Resource the change management effort for success.
- Effectively model integration by including all stakeholders and encouraging "human interoperability." Don't allow people the comfort of continuing to work in their silos.
- Define non-negotiables up front, thereby also defining what is negotiable and can be tailored at a local level.
- Ensure clarity about decision rights, so everyone is clear about who (individuals or committees) has final authority to make which decisions.
- Guard against inundating people with data. Provide them with meaningful information they can understand to help them see how they are doing. Being overwhelmed with data is a distraction and can be confusing.
- Mobilize the executive team and ensure ongoing support for the project.
- Understand the need and actively engage in keeping the organization involved over several years of change, including post go-live.

MISTAKES TO AVOID

Executive sponsors are the glue that holds the project together. This is a critically important role. In the past, executive sponsors have not always recognized the importance of focusing on the people side of EMR deployments. Fortunately, things are changing, and there is increasingly broad recognition that results are dependent on people and that change management is a key success factor. Don't repeat the following mistakes!

- Thinking that change management is someone else's job.
- Adding line items for communication and training to the technical plan and thinking you have change management covered.
- Thinking an EMR implementation is an IT project and letting IT run it.

- Taking the easy way out by thinking of change management and communication as overhead and therefore just a "nice to have" that can be skipped due to resource constraints.
- Believing you can dictate the changes required for a successful EMR implementation, as in "Well, we're installing the boxes, so they will just have to use them." At best, this thinking is naïve.
- Relying on technical or project management staff to take care of the people issues.
- Not showing up! Sponsorship of an EMR implementation takes concerted effort over the long haul. There is personal work required to maintain your own level of commitment throughout the long process. Figure out how you are going to manage yourself, and plan how you will get help—you will probably need it.
- Forgetting the reactions you had when you first considered an EMR implementation a real possibility for your organization. Typically, by the time large numbers of staff hear about the implementation, the senior executives are well past their initial reactions and can become frustrated when staff exhibit normal responses to a proposed change of this magnitude. Remember how you first felt, and give people time to catch up to the point at which you are now.

ENGAGING LEADERS IN THE SPONSOR CASCADE

 Exercise

Here's a simple suggestion executive sponsors can use to engage other leaders in the sponsor cascade:

- Convene a group of direct reports and the next level down to review the EMR vision with discussion.

- Ask the group to identify six to ten things the organization needs to do to make the vision a reality.

- Once the necessary things are identified break the group into small work teams and assign each to develop a plan for their assigned tasks. Mix up the membership of the groups with people from different areas of responsibility to expand thinking and to create alignment.

- The smaller work teams can convene offline to develop plans and then present the plans to the larger group for discussion and feedback.

- Each work team selects a leader to sponsor their plan, integrate it with the EMR project and oversee execution.

Mid-level Sponsors

We haven't said much about middle leaders yet. This does not mean they are not important! In fact, middle leaders are not only critical to implementation success, they are also key to long-term sustainability. If these leaders do not buy in to the vision of electronic medical records; if they do not incorporate new ways of thinking into their daily work; if they do not model the required changes, they will undermine the deployment process and put benefit realization at risk.

Middle leaders are the most overlooked sponsor group. This is of critical importance because sponsorship must be alive and well at the operations level or it is not sustainable. Organizations put a lot of effort into training the front line, and the executives launch and own the EMR effort, but the middle leadership level is often left out of the loop. It is very helpful to put someone in charge of ensuring that middle leaders are supported in making their required transition along with everyone else.

Middle leaders have the same shared sponsor responsibilities listed earlier, in addition to the following:

- Manage up. Report to their executive sponsor escalating issues as needed and ensure that positive and negative reinforcement is applied to their team members appropriately.

Middle leaders must be brought into the EMR process early and must be prepared well if you expect them to take ownership of the vision and the process for getting there.

Supervisor Sponsors

We have stressed the importance of executive and mid-level sponsors. Now we're going to tell you that front-line supervisors are the lynch pin. They own the day-to-day work of their department. Their staff look to them for answers about how jobs will change, how people will be prepared, and what the impact will be to the department, good and bad. With proper preparation and support and adequate time available, supervisors will do much of the heavy lifting to bring their team members along. Here are the keys:

- Train and prepare supervisors early, so they have a chance to understand the technology and know what they are sponsoring.
- Make the EMR implementation a key accountability in supervisor goals and incentive plans to make the EMR priority clear and to give them "skin in the game."
- Engage supervisors in determining the impacts of EMR implementation on their function and people.
- Ensure supervisors play a significant role in workflow harmonization and dress rehearsal design and delivery.
- Have supervisors participate in training with their team members to answer questions about workflow, role changes, scope of practice, policy and procedure, overall implementation process, and coordination with other departments.
- Have supervisors manage up by reporting escalating issues as needed to their mid-level sponsor and ensuring that positive and negative reinforcement are applied appropriately to their team members.

Many studies confirm that the person employees most want to learn about job changes from is their direct supervisor. Think through the questions employees will have during the various stages of the project and ensure that supervisors are prepared to provide the answers. This goes a long way in reducing resistance and increasing feelings of safety, which builds personal confidence and a willingness to participate.

Done well, these overlapping and integrated levels of sponsorship create a strong, self-reinforcing network that supports and guides the organization through change.

FREQUENTLY ASKED QUESTIONS ABOUT SPONSORSHIP

- **How do you know if you have effective sponsorship?**
  - Things work well—issues are escalated and resolved, resources are provided, hard decisions are made, there is role and decision making clarity, and people are held accountable and are openly acknowledged for good performance. The project is meeting its budget and timeline objectives and people are reasonably optimistic that the project will be a success and the future vision achieved. People want to achieve the vision.
- **What do you do if you discover you don't have effective sponsorship?**
  - Engage for commitment. Go back and renegotiate for sponsorship. Be clear about what is needed for success and the risks if strong sponsorship is not present. Discuss the role, find out what the sponsor is willing and able to do, discuss any gaps, determine what kind of support he or she needs, and then reach agreement about what he or she will do going forward. It's a good idea to put the agreement in writing by following up with an e-mail. Part of the agreement should be that you commit to supporting the sponsor with regular meetings to review sponsor performance and plan for next steps—and hold them accountable.
  - Encourage struggling sponsors to assess their own performance against the sponsor role description. Be certain they understand the kinds of support you can provide and encourage them to discuss their needs once they have completed the assessment.
  - Start a sponsor peer group network to provide a means for sponsors from all levels to interact with each other—pose questions, share successful practices **and** mistakes, work together to solve common problems, and make joint decisions. If spread

of homegrown improvements is important to the organization, sponsors openly learning from each other and spreading each others' great ideas will give the concept of continuous improvement some legs.

- Communicate broadly about the sponsor role to help people understand what to go to their sponsors for. The process of being asked to deliver on sponsor accountabilities will reinforce the role, and most sponsors will begin to step up, as most people want to perform well and be successful.
- If all else fails, take your concerns up a level, and discuss the situation with the person who manages the poor performing sponsor.

- **How do you nurture good sponsors when you have them?**
  - Reinforce their good behavior—sponsors are human too and respond to recognition just like everyone else.
  - Coach your sponsors. Start the discussion by asking if you can give them some feedback on what their sponsorship behavior looks like. If sponsorship needs improvement, provide some concrete examples of things to try. And be sure to recognize them for what they are doing well. You don't want them to run every time you ask if you can give feedback.
  - Refer them to the sponsor peer group suggested earlier. Encourage them to share specific things they do that are working and be open about what isn't working to encourage others to talk about what's really on their mind.

- **How do you make the best use of your sponsors?**
  - A great sponsor understands the importance of sponsorship to the success of the project and will be willing to support other sponsors by talking about the role, modeling good sponsor behavior, openly sharing successful and unsuccessful sponsor practices, and actively reinforcing desired behavior.
  - Make it easy for sponsors to deliver needed messages—provide scripts whenever there is something specific to be communicated.
  - Keep sponsors visible. Get them in front of different groups in the organization to reward people, deliver messages, answer questions, and listen.
  - Escalate the hard calls to the right level.

- Encourage sponsors from different constituencies of the organization to partner with each other and model the partnership publicly. There is real impact when leaders co-sponsor across traditional boundaries, such as medical group and management, or union and medical group, or all three together. Try it! Use the project as a way to model doing things differently and see what happens.
- Help sponsors with reinforcement by making it easy for them to reward good behavior and performance, as well as to deliver consequences when needed. Give them easy access to ideas, guidelines, and other resources.
- Actively work with sponsors to ensure continuing commitment and to improve sponsor performance.

- **What if sponsors turn over during the course of the implementation?**
  - Sponsor succession must be planned for. EMR implementation is a multiyear process, and it is likely that you will experience some sponsor turnover. Plan for it, so when it happens, you are prepared and can help your new sponsor get up to speed and performing well quickly.

SPONSORSHIP CHECKLIST

 Checklist

Sponsorship Checklist

❑ The executive sponsor for EMR implementation is on board and has assumed the responsibilities of the role.

❑ Sponsorship for EMR implementation has cascaded from the executive sponsor throughout the leadership levels of the organization down to the front-line supervisors.

❑ All sponsors understand their sponsor role, are prepared to execute well, know what they are expected to deliver and how they will be held accountable.

❑ The EMR implementation is a priority in the organization. Other efforts have been stopped or postponed to enable time and attention to be devoted to electronic medical records.

❑ The executive sponsor takes a long-term view of EMR implementation and benefits realization requirements and ensures adequate financial and human resources are committed to the life of the implementation effort.

❑ The executive sponsor knows that change management starts at his or her door and leads by example to set the tone and direction for the effort.

❑ The executive sponsor is active in reinforcing behaviors required for success and expects the sponsor cascade to model and reinforce at their level.

CHAPTER 4

Organizational Readiness Team

Prescription for Success

In this chapter, we discuss how to structure the technology adoption side of your EMR implementation project. Our recommendation is that you form an organizational readiness team (ORT) comprising all those responsible for people-focused functions. Generally these functions include change management/technology adoption, training, communication, human resources, workforce planning, workflow harmonization, and user lessons learned. And if your organization is unionized, the union engagement function is part of the ORT team as well. It is also helpful to include local champions and subject matter experts (SME) from operations/user communities.

Your organization may refer to people-focused functions by different terms, but the point is still the same—to gather everyone who supports users, as opposed to technology, and get them to integrate and work together. **The organizational readiness team aligns, coordinates, and synchronizes all the people-focused aspects of the project in a way that connects the dots for users.** Do not leave users to do this on their own! Tell one story; begin one narrative about the implementation that builds logically over time in a way that makes sense to users. The organizational readiness components must work together to reach shared goals, integrating and reinforcing each other every step of the way. Do not throw siloed pieces over the wall at users and expect them to do the sense making—you will only create confusion, resentment, and resistance.

Remember, what's important in an EMR implementation is not the system itself but how the new system is used to generate results. The primary objective of the implementation will vary by organization but will revolve around a passion for increasing productivity and taking the waste out, or improving patient safety, or surpassing an externally recognized benchmark, or increasing market share, etc. The objective is to install the EMR **only** as it is a required step, a key enabler that makes achievement of the primary objective possible. Don't lose sight of this perspective in the effort it takes to install the system. Make the passion clear and explicit.

ORGANIZATIONAL READINESS TEAM DEFINED

We use the term *organizational readiness* with system implementation projects because it ties together all the people-focused aspects and works well across all phases of the project. The purpose of the ORT is to lead and manage the cultural, behavioral, and operational changes that need to take place, so that users are willing and able to successfully transition to the future state. The ORT works collaboratively to develop realistic plans to prepare people and get them involved in **how** the implementation will be done.

For a large organization, in which there may be local ORTs in addition to a corporate level ORT for the project, a successful practice is to connect these teams in a network. The larger team associated with the corporate office convenes and facilitates the network, providing opportunities for sharing learnings, successful practices, tools and techniques, and, in some cases, resources. This practice speeds learning, reduces variation, and makes the entire organizational readiness effort more efficient and effective. If you are large enough, subject matter areas may want to form sub-teams as well. This means you might have a training sub-team (one for communication for example) in addition to the larger network that all people-focused staff participate in.

Example: In one large organization, the training leads from the various locations started the practice of a biweekly conference call. At first the participants didn't say much, few questions were asked, and most of the time was spent on updates delivered by the corporate office. But when a couple of people from outlying areas began asking for help with issues, other people offered suggestions, and trust began to grow. Soon this training conference call had a reputation as the place for trainers to be. Many more people joined and what once was a short call with a few people and not much significant content became the problem-solving body for the entire training function for the project. Trainers were united; they shared resources, tools, and learnings across traditional organizational boundaries, and the users were the beneficiaries.

Key Point

Organizational Readiness Team Objectives

- Define strategy, structure and vision for people-focused work.

- Assess the organizational history of success or failure with change efforts and how this influences people's thinking.

- Collaborate across organizational boundaries—work together.

- Develop overall people readiness plan and tools. Integrate ORT milestones with the technical plan.

- Develop common understanding of user readiness for each phase of the project.

- Provide clarity—connect the dots for users, create one story.

- Sequence activities in a way that is logical for users and builds over time.

- Coordinate resources across the organization.

- Ensure success for each user by developing willingness and ability—address issues of both hearts and minds.

- Create an environment that supports and reinforces users in moving to the future state.

- Bring people together through peer groups and conferences.

- Learn as you go, and instill a continuous learning culture.

PROJECT PHASES

There are generally five main project phases for an EMR implementation. The project begins with the initial planning phase and transitions through implementation, stabilization, optimization and finally benefit realization. The full project life cycle is introduced in Figure 4-1 and broken out in steps in Figures 4-2 through 4-6, but the focus of this book is predominantly on preparing people for implementation. Although we do not discuss the later phases in depth, the lessons we present will guide you in establishing the appropriate context and platform for a seamless and successful journey to benefit realization.

Figure 4-1: Project Life Cycle

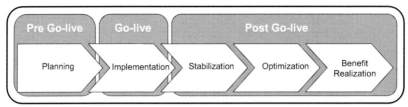

It is important to note that although we discuss the project phases as if they are discrete, they are in fact overlapping to some degree. If you work in a large organization, different phases may be running simultaneously in different locations. This adds complexity, but if you are aware of it, the situation is easier to manage.

Planning

During the planning phase (see Figure 4-2), the ORT forms, gathers resources, develops strategy, and plans to prepare people and the organization for implementation/go-live. At a high level, the following is involved:

- Becoming a sponsored, recognized, legitimate part of the EMR project charter and implementation team.
- Obtaining budget, staff commitments, and other resources.
- Spelling out ORT team roles and responsibilities.
- Conducting an organizational implementation history assessment to understand the organizational history with change efforts and how that currently influences people's thinking about the EMR project. Factor findings into the ORT strategy and workplan.
- Developing the organizational readiness strategy and approach for the project.
- Developing a detailed ORT workplan for the implementation phase.
- Integrating ORT workplan milestones with the technical workplan.
- Conducting an operational and job impact assessment to determine the points at which job impacts are greatest and, at a high level, what the changes are and whether the changes will result in job loss and/or significant need for retraining.

Figure 4-2: Planning Phase of Project Life Cycle

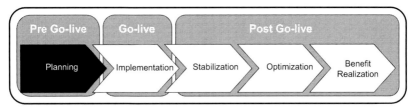

- Developing and beginning to implement realistic plans to prepare people (willingness and ability) for go-live—includes sponsor development strategy, stakeholder identification and management plan, training model and plan, communication plan, managing resistance strategy, assessing job impact, etc. Union engagement begins too, when needed, as does engagement with operations areas.

Implementation

Depending on the size of your organization, the implementation process (see Figure 4-3) could mean a few events happening over a relatively short period or it could mean many go-lives happening over the course of a few years. Factors that influence this phase include the number of facilities you have, whether the organization favors a "big bang" or a phased implementation approach, and the number and type of applications being implemented as part of your EMR deployment.

The implementation phase is the period when the system is launched and users begin to use the system on the job with real patients for the first time. This is a period of much excitement for some and much anxiety for others. Users are faced with trying to remember everything they learned prior to go-live and applying it in real life situ-

Figure 4-3: Implementation Phase of Project Life Cycle

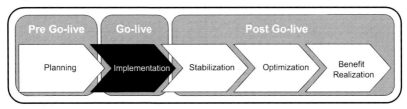

ations. This can be overwhelming, scary, and intimidating. During the implementation phase, the ORT focuses on ensuring that users can get through their day, working closely with the support teams and sponsors to ensure that users feel supported and that the environment continues to reinforce desired behaviors.

The following are key ORT work items during the implementation phase:

- Delivering training and ensuring the "sandbox" (practice site), Web-based training modules, job aides, and other learning options are current, effective and readily available.
- Communication is fully engaged in ensuring that users, sponsors, and project team members know what they need to know when they need to know it. Feedback loops are active, and comments and questions are responded to in a timely manner.
- Successes are celebrated, and individuals and teams are recognized for great performance and achievement of milestones.
- Plans for managing anticipated job losses are put in place.
- Unions are actively involved to ensure members are well-supported to be successful in the transition and that the changes are implemented according to contract terms.
- User lessons learned activities begin with the first go-lives. Learnings are shared broadly and recommended improvements are made to subsequent go-lives.
- Sponsors continue to be coached and supported to perform their roles well.

Though the focus of this book is on planning and implementation, we provide a short review of stabilization, optimization, and benefits realization here (see Figures 4-4 through 4-6) to provide an overall picture of the end-to-end process.

Stabilization

As you can imagine, the EMR implementation can be overwhelming for many users and can feel like a whirlwind of new experiences. Users are busy trying to apply what they can remember from training and team readiness sessions (discussed in Chapter 9, Implementation Readiness). And now that the system is becoming part of the new daily routine, users begin to see what works and what doesn't work with the

Figure 4-4: Stabilization Phase of Project Life Cycle

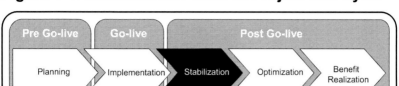

overall operational flow. Teams revisit decisions about workflows that were made before go-live and begin to make necessary adjustments to increase efficiencies on their units (see Figure 4-4).

Stabilization is the time when the organization should pause to make sure users have a chance to digest the experience and assimilate the many changes that are taking place. Unfortunately, too many organizations become anxious and make the mistake of jumping to the next project phase, optimization, without ensuring users are comfortable in their roles, feel well supported, and are catching on to the new system.

Use this important post-live time to truly stabilize your operations! Users are a bit distracted with the changes that have taken place and are at a point when they need the space to sort out their new life with an EMR. They are still trying to just get through their work day and are not ready for additional changes and/or technology enhancements just yet. Allow users the time to get their feet solidly on the ground, cement their new learning, and develop confidence before moving on. Jumping to optimization too quickly can cause a costly setback, which will delay the entire process.

Stabilization doesn't necessarily need to be long and drawn out, but it is important to note that individual differences begin to surface again during this phase. There is a big divide in user effectiveness with the EMR at this point. Early adopters want to move forward and make enhancements to the system, while other users are trying to just catch their breath and assimilate everything that is happening. This scenario can be tricky to manage, but the biggest mistake is forging ahead without doing the work required to create a more or less level playing field by addressing individual skill differences. Most users do not learn more about the system post-live unless there is an intervention. **Do**

not assume they will eventually catch up on their own! If you don't address the skill variation issue during stabilization, the divide will deepen with slow and average users falling farther and farther behind the early adopters.

During the planning phase when you develop, document and resource the project, a key success factor is planning for a solid stabilization period. After everything you will go through to implement, it doesn't make sense to put the project at risk by not fully addressing post-live needs before pressing on.

During stabilization the ORT continues to support users in settling into a routine using the system, helps with adjustments to roles and workflows, ensures user skills are assessed, and provides additional training or coaching required to attain the expected level of proficiency. User lessons learned are responded to and documented for future reference. Reinforcement of desired behaviors continues and implementation successes are celebrated.

Optimization

There is a fine distinction between the stabilization and optimization phases. Typically, organizations combine the phases and view stabilization as a subset of optimization. In a sense, stabilization is a span of time (short or long) during which the organization can take a deep breath, regroup, and ensure everyone is still on the same page before forging ahead into more significant change. The stabilization phase (see Figure 4-4) is analogous to the act of refueling your car and making brief pit stops during a vacation before continuing the family road trip across country. A car can only travel so far with one tank of gas, and everyone knows that vacations are no fun when everyone is cranky, hungry, and sick of being in the car. Users need the same consideration because burnout and fatigue can compromise the willingness to withstand subsequent change efforts.

Many say that optimization (see Figure 4-5) is the place where the action happens. If the stabilization phase has gone well, users are now becoming comfortable with their new roles and routines and are ready to become more efficient in using the system. This is what organizations strive for—efficient use can lead to faster returns on this significant investment. Unfortunately, just as with stabilization, organizations

Figure 4-5: Optimization Phase of Project Life Cycle

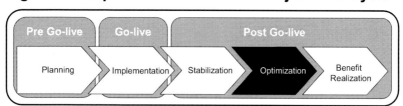

tend to rush through optimization trying to get to benefit realization, and this can actually delay achieving the goal.

One of the biggest mistakes organizations make at this stage is to declare victory too early and reassign project resources, discounting the need for an ongoing people-focused strategy. The optimization phase is an important and exciting part of the journey, but it requires fully engaged and prepared users. Just as users needed preparation for implementation, they need further preparation if they are to grow into becoming truly proficient. Developing proficiency requires targeted training, workflow improvements, support, and continued leadership. Significant work must take place during this phase, and there are many successful practices from which lessons may be learned. For now, as we said earlier, remember that your organization will be primed for a successful optimization phase only when an appropriate context for change and learning is established during the planning and implementation phases.

Organizational Readiness Team Role in Optimization

- Work with executives and project leads to develop and run reports to gauge user performance toward operational and clinical targets.

- Conduct user proficiency assessments to surface user skill gaps and uncover broken workflows.

- Partner with the training and support teams to develop targeted and timely interventions to increase proficiency.

- Ensure training and support is role-based and department-specific.

- Develop programs and tools to increase operational efficiencies, partnering with key stakeholder groups such as quality services, medical group, management and labor.

- Coach and mentor front-line leaders in monitoring performance and providing the tools and resources needed to assess process improvements.

- Obtain lessons learned from across the organization and spread best practice approaches.

Benefit Realization

Benefit realization (see Figure 4-6) is the grand prize for successfully moving your organization through the phases of the project life cycle. This is where desired outcomes become a reality and the organization begins to see improvements in revenue capture, patient safety, patient satisfaction, work/life balance, internal efficiencies, and so forth.

At this point, the role of the ORT is to continue developing and delivering effective optimization programs to enhance user performance, spread successful practices and ensure teams across all departments and facilities are learning from each other and incorporating the most effective new ways of doing things.

Figure 4-6: Benefit Realization Phase of Project Life Cycle

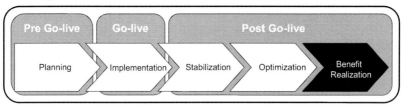

Figure 4-7: Organizational Readiness Team Structure

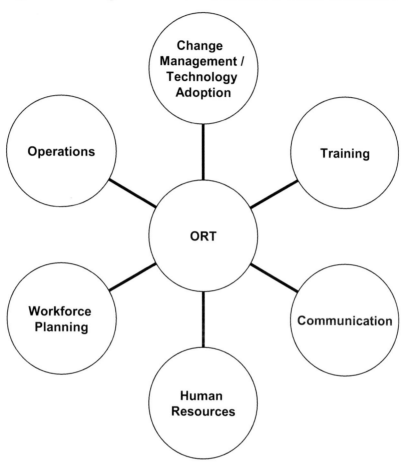

ORGANIZATIONAL READINESS TEAM

Each subject matter area represented on the ORT performs a different role in preparing individuals and the organization to successfully make the changes required by the EMR implementation. But it is important to remember that the elements of organizational readiness are interdependent and reinforcing. They are most effective when aligned, coordinated, and synchronized.

When forming the ORT (see Figure 4-7), select the best people you have, not those that you can do without. For a project with this much importance to the organization, you need the best and the brightest.

Change Management/Technology Adoption

Change management typically leads the organizational readiness team, ensuring the coordination, integration, and alignment of all the people-focused work. Change management/technology adoption ensures that team members are embracing a systems perspective and are working in concert to weave a supportive organizational fabric (culture) for successful change. Change management/technology adoption also leads overall sponsor support; stakeholder management; and political, interpersonal and team development issue resolution.

Training

Effective training prepares users to do their job in the new world of electronic medical records. It is much more than just software feature/function training. Using the system effectively is part of it, but users also need to understand how the new system fits into their job, including orientation to new workflows; policies; and procedures; and anything else that changes because of the EMR implementation.

Communication

The role and purpose of communication supporting an EMR implementation is discussed in Chapter 6, the Communication chapter. The overarching goal is to successfully drive behavior change. Communication helps set the tone for the project, delivers information in a timely and appropriate manner, and solicits and responds to feedback about the project.

Human Resources

Human resource involvement includes:
- Adjusting job descriptions, titles, and reporting structures as appropriate.
- Working with workforce planning to gauge job impact from the EMR implementation and managing position eliminations, reassignments, and retirements, as indicated.
- Revising recruitment/hiring criteria to reflect new EMR requirements.
- Aligning incentives to reinforce the behavior changes and performance outcomes required in the new EMR world.

Workforce Planning

We call out workforce planning separately because it is such an important component of an EMR implementation. If any positions will be eliminated due to the EMR implementation, the sooner this is known the better. Workforce planning identifies the impacted roles and determines how the position elimination process will be managed. In some cases eliminated staff can be trained to fill new roles. Figure out all the details well before you need to give notice. The same goes for potential reassignments and retirements. All of these situations are complex processes, especially if you are unionized. Don't wait until the last minute! Treat employees with respect by doing your very best for them in this difficult situation.

✓ Lesson Learned

Not everyone will survive the transition to EMRs. Anticipate that roughly 5% will leave the organization. To plan for this, you need a robust, proactive workforce planning effort.

Operational Representatives

If you are unionized, we can't stress enough the importance of early and frequent engagement with unions. This happens at three levels:

- **Union leadership.** Many of these people are employed by the union, not the healthcare organization.
- **Represented employees.** These are the people in your organization that belong to a union and are subject to the stipulations of the bargaining contract that covers them.
- **Represented employees with union leadership roles.** Among the ranks of represented employees, there are generally leadership roles, such as steward and contract specialist. People in these roles are employed by the healthcare organization, and their union leadership responsibilities are in addition to their day-to-day job responsibilities.

> **Lesson Learned**
>
> If you are unionized, engage union leaders early and often! Don't wait. Get them involved in the project from the beginning.

Operational representatives do not need to attend every planning session, but they are integral to the overall success of the development and execution of the technology adoption program. Operational representatives can include union partners, physicians, nurses, clinical supervisors, and other stakeholders depending on the exact EMR application you are implementing. For some organizations, the EMR is fully integrated, and thus it is important to include representatives from many different groups within the organization. We cover four important operational groups here: unions, physicians, local champions and super users. (Sponsors, mid-level managers and front-line supervisors are covered in Chapter 3 on Sponsorship.)

UNION ENGAGEMENT FOR SUCCESSFUL EMR IMPLEMENTATION

Marie Hamilton, RN, Kaiser Permanente, explains, "Unions recognize that the decision to implement an EMR is an organizational business decision and do not expect to be involved in the decision-making process. But after the decision is made, organizational leaders should consider early communication to union leaders with a request for their support and sponsorship. Engaging union leaders at the highest level of planning creates an environment of trust and collaboration, decreases resistance, facilitates sponsorship and engagement at all levels and is essential to ensuring a smooth implementation and transition for users. Success of the implementation becomes a shared accountability.

Once union leaders are committed to sponsorship, involving them in the development of the business case engages union leaders in return on investment expectations. This is a great opportunity for union and management to understand the goals and each others' roles and responsibilities. Together they can begin planning strategies and approaches to achieve the required outcomes. Involvement at this level will also facilitate early discussion about the bargaining process, which will be required to address the changes in working conditions that are inherent in technology implementation of this magnitude.

When administrators and managers acknowledge the expertise of users, the IT team and union leaders will be empowered to develop engagement strategies that maximize the knowledge and expertise of both the IT and provider sides of the equation. Front-line workers want to be active participants from beginning discussions to designing of workflows that address the realities of day-to-day operations. Combining IT expertise with user knowledge and credibility helps to minimize costly mistakes that result from inefficient processes and potentially dangerous workarounds.

Users can assist IT to assess skill gaps by conducting skills assessments in a safe environment. The results will provide accurate information to inform training needs. Users are often the best resource to deliver peer training with an IT partner."

Hamilton summarizes her thoughts in the following Union Perspective.

Union Perspective

- Involve union leaders early, and ask them to be sponsors.

- Involve union leaders in creation of the business case.

- Create a venue for open dialogue to address changes requiring bargaining, so there are no surprises (or grievances).

- Work with unions to create a structure for user participation at all levels of implementation, utilizing them as subject matter experts.

- Training will be more successful if designed and delivered by a team of IT trainers and users working together.

- Utilize front-line staff as expert support during go-live. Staff respond better and feel less stressed when their peers who fully understand the work help them through the process. An added bonus is that the peer support staff return to work and continue to help their team members through the transition.

- Unions want to know that they have a real decision-making voice in the process which so profoundly affects them. By meaningfully engaging and acknowledging their contributions, the transition will be smoother for everyone. The organization, the union and most of all, the patients will benefit.

Marie Hamilton, RN
Kaiser Permanente
Oregon Federation of Nurses and Health Professionals
Healthcare Information Technology Committee, AFT Healthcare

PHYSICIANS

Physicians are critically important in the planning process as well. As one physician comments:

Physician Perspective

Engagement, engagement, engagement!

I cannot stress this enough. Physicians must be engaged throughout the whole project including decision making, design, testing, support and implementation. The project team must consider the impact decisions have on workflows and user work/life balance. Without physicians at the table, the technology will fail at supporting daily operations and lead to many problems and inefficiencies down the road.

Nabil Chehade, MD, MSBS, CPC
Director, Medical Informatics
Regional Chief of Urology
KP HealthConnect Regional Physician Lead
Kaiser Permanente Medical Group

LOCAL CHAMPIONS

 Key Tip

Local champions are your best friends.

Because all change is local, the people receiving the new technology should drive the change, with IT as the enabler. Trusted peer-to-peer influence is one of the most effective ways of moving change forward, or stopping it, which makes informal local leaders extremely valuable when effectively used. We strongly recommend that you identify, train, and get local champions involved early in the process. They will be needed from any areas that will experience significant impact from the EMR implementation.

It is important to choose the right people for this role. When we say *local champion,* we mean a local, informal opinion leader. Informal leaders may or may not also be formal leaders with titles. In most cases, they are not, and you will need to look further than the organization chart to find them. The easiest way to do this is to ask around. Ask people the following questions:

- Who does everyone listen to when an important decision needs to be made?
- Who does the whole department turn to for advice on an issue or to solve a problem?
- Who is highly respected and trustworthy?
- Who do people want representing the department on committees or project teams?

When you hear the same names repeatedly, you will know who the informal leaders are. Choose well. On a technology project, it is tempting to look for the people who are technically savvy. Unfortunately, though they may be easier to identify and are clearly interested in technology, technically skilled people generally do not make good local champions. The reason is that, for areas in which most people's computer skills are average or below, the "geeks" are not seen as representative of the team. Their ability to learn to use new technology is not seen as proof that anyone else will ever be able to learn it.

Find other roles for the technically skilled people, and choose local champions that can truly represent their peers, both in content and technical ability. Let the technology experts on the project team represent the technical considerations. The local champions provide the knowledge of the day to day work in their functional areas. In our experience, the best ideas and solutions are developed when technical and content experts work together.

The following selection criteria for local champions will help you identify the right people. **Local champions must:**

- Be social influencers who are thought/opinion leaders with informal power.
- Be the diplomats who translate reality back and forth between the project team and their department. They carry messages with integrity and honesty.
- Be able to get the right people together to reach decisions.
- Involve team members; find the right roles to get the best from them and keep them motivated.
- Persevere!
- Give and receive feedback well.

- Be trustworthy, ethical, credible, and respected.
- Be willing to serve the team; be collaborative by nature.
- Have a positive outlook.
- Have high credibility with sponsors.
- Be willing and able to model the expected changes (role, workflow, etc.)—learn it first, then model and teach it to others. When team members see local champions learn, they believe they can learn too.

What is the role of local champions? Essentially they represent the interests of their functional area and serve as conduits for information. They participate in project meetings, representing their department interests/needs, and then bring information back. They answer questions from team members and take concerns about the implementation of the project for resolution. The objective is to ensure the local needs are reflected in the project planning and that project information is delivered and reinforced by respected, trusted team members.

An advantage of using local champions is that it is a way to get input from many through the voices of a few. Great local champions enable team members to participate and influence the EMR project through representation. This allows for more involvement without overburdening the project or the department—a nice balance.

Local champion success factors:
- Have a clear method for identifying informal leaders.
- Clearly define the local champion role.
- Select for credibility and ability to influence peers, not on availability or technical skill. Teach the required technical skills.
- Establish a training model for champion skill development and provide EMR software training early.
- Give local champions meaningful tasks to obtain their buy-in and maintain their engagement and commitment to the project. Meaningful work includes implementation planning, system demonstrations, training, workflow redesign, issue resolution, etc.
- Leverage their social relationships to gain buy-in across their department and professional community.
- Use local champions to help identify resistance and determine how best to manage it.

- Make the local champion role part of the job. Reduce other responsibilities enough for people to perform the role effectively.

SUPER USERS

Super users can also be local champions, but they are not necessarily. The super user role is local and is generally assigned to front-line team members who want to develop deep knowledge of the system for the primary purpose of training and troubleshooting on their unit. Super users are part of the on-the-ground support network and in our view, the role should remain in place for the life of the EMR.

To make the best use of super users, expand the role to include ongoing participation with IT in system enhancements and issue resolution. People who have deep functional knowledge and are highly skilled at using the system to do the daily work are invaluable. Form a network of super users; bring them together quarterly to share learnings, spread successful practices and problem-solve. This is a huge step in moving the EMR from a project to a fully integrated tool for operations.

Both super users and local champions play an important role in helping their team members learn and adjust to the new system. The old adage "see one, do one, teach one" fits well here. Super users and champions learn new things with the system and with workflows, which they teach others. Being coached by a trusted colleague makes a big difference to people who are frustrated or fearful. Trying something new with supportive supervision and immediate feedback is powerful—people learn and build confidence. And the medical assistant who learns a new skill and then teaches it to a colleague cements the skill for himself or herself. (See one, do one, teach one.)

Super users must have part of their role devoted to this responsibility. They need to participate in project and super user meetings, attend training, and deliver training and support in their department. This will not happen if they are completely tied to patient care or to a business responsibility. Find the right people and free a portion of their time, so they can assume project responsibilities on an ongoing basis.

Checklist

Organizational Readiness Team Checklist

❑ Form an organizational readiness team (ORT) comprised of all people-focused functions.

❑ Connect local and corporate level ORT in a network for collaboration, successful practice and lessons learned spread, problem solving, and resource and tool sharing.

❑ Ensure the elements of organizational readiness are interdependent and reinforcing. They are most effective when aligned, coordinated and synchronized.

❑ Conduct user lessons learned after at least the first go-live events for each application. Use the lessons to improve subsequent go-lives. Circle back to users who participated in the lessons to let them know how their input contributed to improvement.

❑ If you are unionized, engage union leaders early and often. Don't wait.

❑ Identify, engage, train and fully utilize local champions to communicate with and influence their peers, and to inform the project team of local needs and realities.

❑ Form a network of highly trained super users as part of on-the-ground support. Use them to handle training and other issues at the department level.

Willingness—
Building Commitment

CHAPTER 5

Stakeholder Management

They must have skin in the game.

Identifying and understanding stakeholders is a critical early step in organizational readiness work. Stakeholder identification takes commitment and time—you may be tempted to gloss over it or not do it at all. But remember that knowing who your stakeholders are and what makes them tick informs all the people-focused areas of the project and some of the technical areas as well. It is worth the effort and will pay big dividends when done well.

STAKEHOLDER DEFINITION

The term *stakeholders* refers to the groups that will be impacted by the EMR implementation and whose participation or support is needed to reach the goal. This means everyone who has a stake of some kind in the changes that will occur as the organization begins to use EMRs. Stakeholders can be departments, committees, or functional areas. They can also be employees, patients, and companies that do business with your organization. The point is to think this through carefully to identify everyone who has a stake in the changes that will occur.

As a point of clarification, generally speaking, stakeholders are groups of people and sponsors are individuals. Please see Chapter 3 on Sponsorship for more information on sponsors and their responsibilities.

THE IMPORTANCE OF STAKEHOLDER IDENTIFICATION, ENGAGEMENT, AND MANAGEMENT

Technology adoption is a completely people-focused endeavor. You cannot succeed at it unless you really understand the people you are supporting—who they are, the degree of impact they are facing, their day-to-day reality, their concerns and hopes, and how they are reacting to the change at any given point. This knowledge and the ability to successfully influence stakeholders to move from where they are to where you want them to be is a very significant contribution. Together, skilled change management/technology adoption professionals working in close collaboration with other people-focused partners deliver the user readiness on which the success of an EMR implementation depends.

Three Steps of Stakeholder Management

1. The first requirement in stakeholder management is to **identify** all groups and individuals, inside and outside the organization, who will be affected by the EMR implementation. This includes identification of sponsors. The section on Stakeholder/Sponsor Identification and Mapping that follows describes a process you can use to accomplish this task.

2. Once your stakeholders are identified, your second step will be to create a strategy and a plan to **engage** them in the implementation process based on what you know about them. Build your knowledge and establish a relationship as a trusted partner—get out in their world, watch what happens and listen. There is nothing more valuable than the deep understanding you gain from this activity. It is a means of correctly identifying how and to what extent different groups are impacted. This helps you understand what each stands to gain or lose and what they must do differently to succeed in the EMR implementation. The following are key questions to ask to gather the information you need:
   - What problems or issues do you have with the way things are currently done?
   - How would you improve the situation if you were in charge?

- What potential opportunities do you see with the EMR implementation?
- How much of an impact do you think the implementation will have on your department?
- What are you most concerned about with the EMR implementation?
- What are the most effective ways to get information out to your department?
- What is the best way for you to provide feedback to the project?
- Who else in your department should I talk to about the EMR implementation?

3. The third step is ongoing stakeholder **management.** This is the design and implementation of strategies to support and move stakeholders forward. It requires that you pay attention to how stakeholders are behaving and what they are saying in order to understand what their needs are at any given point. If you know them and you know at what point they are in the change process, you can provide just what they need when they need it. Some stakeholder groups will need minimal levels of information periodically, and others will need to be directly involved in the project. You must know the difference on the continuum, from information only to direct involvement to decision making.

Key Tip

Understanding stakeholder needs is a means of identifying dissatisfaction. Dissatisfaction is a change enabler.

STAKEHOLDER/SPONSOR IDENTIFICATION AND MAPPING

A comprehensive stakeholder/sponsor map is an important foundational building block in an EMR implementation. The identification and mapping process is best conducted early in the project, as stakeholder identification is a prerequisite to many other aspects of the implementation, such as:

- **Communication**—Stakeholders are the audiences with whom you communicate.
- **Training**—Identifying stakeholder groups is the first step in identifying roles, and this drives user-centric curriculum.
- **Reinforcement**—Reinforcement has the most impact when it is tailored to specific individuals and groups.
- **Sponsorship**—The stakeholder map is an important tool in identifying sponsors.
- **Organizational Readiness Team**—The stakeholder map helps identify areas where super users and local champions are needed.
- **Technical considerations**—Different stakeholders may need different kinds of equipment or devices; or the EMR may interface with existing applications, etc.

You can see that the stakeholder/sponsor map plays an important role in EMR implementation. It is admittedly a lot of work to compile, but it is an investment well made. The map will serve many uses in the project and will most likely have much broader organizational application. A good stakeholder map lends clarity to organizational structure, shows linkages across the organization, and very importantly, helps the project team understand who the customers of the implementation are, both inside and outside the organization.

The first step is to fully identify all the people and groups in your organization who will be impacted by the EMR implementation. Cast a wide net when you do this. These are the audiences you will communicate with, influence, and train during the project. It is easy to overlook groups who need to be informed or involved that might not be readily apparent. Here's an example:

A few years ago at one organization, no one thought to engage with the people who cleaned the building at night to help them understand how the EMR implementation would impact their work. Many of the individuals responsible for cleaning the equipment had no computer experience, so they did not know how to clean the machines. Later, when problems with keyboards were surfacing, it was discovered that some individuals were spraying the keyboards with liquid cleaner. The oversight of not defining Environmental Services as a stakeholder in the project cost the organization some unbudgeted expense in replacing keyboards.

So the first rule of thumb is to identify *everyone* who is impacted, regardless of degree of impact. Start with your internal groups but remember to include external groups too, such as patients, vendors, referring physicians, legal counsel—anyone who may have a need to know something at some point in the project. It will take more time to be thorough in this effort but it will pay off in the long run. It's a case of slowing down now to go fast later.

Refer to your EMR case for change and vision to help you think about who will be impacted by the change. Then complete the following exercise to identify stakeholders and build a stakeholder map. It's not high tech, but it is a flexible process and it works.

Stakeholder/Sponsor Identification Exercise

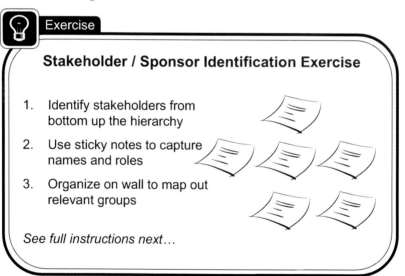

EXERCISE INSTRUCTIONS

❑ Gather a small group of people who have insight into how the EMR implementation will impact the organization. Bring sticky notes and pens and organization charts if you have them.

❑ Begin by looking inside your organization. Where you look first will depend on how large your organization is and how it is structured. To simplify this process description, let's assume you are beginning with a focus on one hospital. If your organization is large and has multiple regions and facilities, you will need to repeat this process for each area or location that will be impacted.

❑ Start by identifying all the people, areas, and groups at the lowest level of the hospital that will be impacted by the applications you will be implementing.

❑ For each person or group that you identify, write the name on a sticky note and attach it to the wall, a white board, or large sheets of paper.

❑ Next, using a different color sticky note, identify the managers for each person or group and place their names above the names already on the wall.

❑ Continue this process, working your way up the organization until you have gone as high as needed. For an EMR implementation, this will be all the way to the executive suite of the hospital. Your chart will look like a typical organizational chart.

❑ Once you have the chart put together, identify managers and other leaders who will be sponsors of the implementation. The sponsorship cascade usually reflects the reporting structure in an organization. Starting at the top, sponsorship flows down the successive levels until you reach front-line management.

❑ Once you have completed this process for the obvious internal people and departments, think about other areas of the hospital that your identified stakeholders interface with or impact. Add these areas to the chart.

❑ The next step is to think outside of the hospital to identify other parts of the healthcare system (if your organization is larger than one hospital), as well as people and groups that are not part of your organization, such as vendors, patients, etc., who will be impacted.

❑ When you think you have identified all impacted parties, take a careful look at the map and adjust the sticky notes as needed. Groups that naturally fit together due to profession, function, customer set, or reporting structure are stakeholder groups. They run both up and down, as well as across the hospital. For example, a nurse is a member of both her medical-surgical unit stakeholder group and her broader hospital-wide nursing stakeholder group. Depending on complexity you may need more than one map to fully paint the picture.

❏ The final step is to create a soft version of the map(s), using a software application. Once this has been done, you can easily share the document with others to get their input. Make final changes as needed.

Again, the reason for going to all the trouble to create a stakeholder map is to inform the project team. Knowing who the stakeholders are allows you to develop understanding of their perspective and needs so that you can be targeted and specific in your plans and actions. It is impossible to be role-specific and user-centric if you don't know who these people are!

Though this process may seem daunting, it is well worth the effort. You don't have to get it all done in one sitting; in fact, we've never seen that happen. It takes multiple iterations to complete because many people need to contribute their knowledge. It is a fascinating process, and you will learn a lot as you work through it.

Key Tip

Don't let the minutiae of stakeholder mapping slow you down. Do the best you can to get started. Once you have a map at least partially completed, identify the top five (or so) most impacted groups and focus on getting to know them first. Fill in more stakeholders and details as they become known.

STAKEHOLDER ENGAGEMENT
AND MANAGEMENT

> **" " Quote**
>
> "Coming together is a beginning; keeping together is progress; working together is success."
>
> - Henry Ford

Once you have a stakeholder map, you can begin to plan how you will engage your stakeholders in the process of EMR implementation and how you will help manage their experience with the many changes that will impact them.

It's important to identify those stakeholders who are most critical in the process. These will obviously be groups that will experience the greatest degree of change. But you should also identify groups or individuals who can positively or negatively impact the project. On the positive side, these include potential super users, local informal opinion leaders, those who have a lot to gain, and anyone with positive experience with other change efforts. On the more negative side, look for the resisters, those who stand to lose a lot, and anyone with past negative experience with organizational change.

Getting stakeholders involved in the process is a way of developing acceptance and buy-in and giving them a say in *how* the implementation will be handled. When people have an opportunity to participate in and influence decisions that affect them, the process becomes less about something being done to them and more about something being done with them.

Next are two tools you can use to assess the status of your various stakeholders. Both of these methods are valuable ways of thinking about where people currently are and what they are experiencing at given points during the implementation. This knowledge is invaluable in formulating communication pieces, addressing resistance, applying effective interventions, identifying people who can be of assistance, and heading off problems—all aspects of the ORT role.

Figure 5-1: Bell Curve

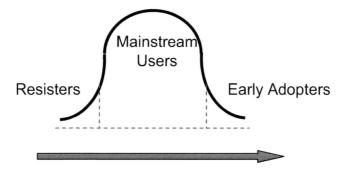

Use these two tools throughout the project to inform your ongoing stakeholder management process.

The Bell Curve

This is a simple process (see Figure 5-1) in which you determine at a high level at what point individuals/groups fall into readiness categories of early adopters, mainstream users, or resisters. There are a variety of terms used to define each of these states, and some models break it down into five or seven states. To keep this simple, we will use three. Please see the example featured above.

Your task is to identify the points at which key individuals or groups are on the bell curve. Their status will change over the course of the project, so you will want to revisit this on an as-needed basis. Remember, the purpose of doing this exercise is that it will provide you with insights into why people are doing what they are doing so you can figure out what you can do to effectively and respectfully support them in moving forward. The objective is to move resisters to mainstream status, while leveraging the expertise of the early adopters. If you can get the middle to move over, they generally bring the resisters with them.

Here is some general information about the characteristics of each of the three categories of adoption readiness and some things you can do for each group.

EARLY ADOPTERS

These are the people who jump on early, love the concept of an EMR, wanted it yesterday, and in fact may be ahead of some people on the project team. They tend to have a positive attitude about change but can become disgruntled if they think the project isn't executing correctly. Early EMR adopters tend to be highly computer literate and high users of technology in their personal lives. You may want to select them for roles on the project, and there are many things they can do to contribute. But they are not suitable candidates for local champion roles because rank and file users do not always relate to them. This group can benefit from:

- Being productively involved in the implementation project in a way that leverages their technical expertise.
- Being trained early, so they can work on groups to help think through elements, such as workflow changes, training scenarios, testing, and developing job aides.
- Early adopters who are not viewed as "propeller heads" and who are good teachers make excellent demonstrators, trainers, and super users.
- Early adopters who figure out how the system can work for them (instead of the other way around) can make a significant contribution. Find them!

MAINSTREAM USERS

This group, generally speaking, will survive (and even thrive) the transition to the EMR if they are provided with appropriate information, training, and support. They are more cautious than the early adopters but they do not tend toward negativity. They just want to know what's going on, what's happening to them, and how they will be supported to succeed. They tend to be comfortable with change and may actually be very open-minded and interested in new technology. They may or may not have good typing and computer skills. This group can benefit from building confidence through:

- Early demonstrations of the software and a chance to talk to respected, informed early adopters about how the system will work and what the anticipated benefits are.

- Hearing from respected local opinion leaders about how the implementation will be handled, what the anticipated difficulties might be, and that they can learn the system and be successful!
- Early typing and computer skill assessment, with easily accessible courses available for skill development prior to system training.
- Opportunities to ask questions and get credible answers to their concerns.

RESISTERS

This group of people tends to believe they have a lot to lose in the EMR implementation. Many of them don't like change in general, and one as sweeping as an EMR is particularly unsettling. They may have poor or non-existent computer and typing skills and tend to be limited users of technology at home. You may have some who are computer literate but are resistant because they do not believe the EMR product the organization is implementing is good enough. This group can benefit from overcoming concerns through:

- One-on-one early demonstration of the software and a chance to ask questions about their concerns.
- Detailed descriptions of how they will be supported through the transition.
- Chances to talk to peers from other organizations or areas that have been through the transition and are doing well and to see the benefits first-hand.
- Honest talk. Don't sugar-coat or oversell.
- Early typing and computer skill assessment, with easily accessible courses available for skill development prior to system training.
- Opportunities to express their misgivings (surfacing resistance) and be heard.
- For some, becoming directly involved in the project is a great thing. When influential resisters are converted to advocates, they can be very vocal and persuasive with their peers.

The Change Curve

The change curve presents a high-level overview of the process people go through when moving through change. It is straightforward and

Figure 5-2: Change Curve

(From IMA. *Accelerating Implementation Methodology (AIM)*; 2009. www.imaworldwide.com.[3] Used by permission.)

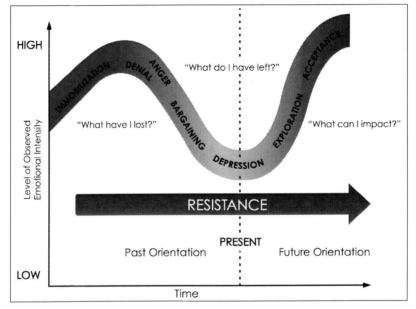

easy to understand. You will probably recognize your own experiences with change when you look at the curve.

When you see the change process as a normal and predictable human experience it reduces anxiety associated with change. Understanding the curve helps you understand yourself and this makes it easier to manage your own reactions to change. Understanding the curve also helps you be much more effective at supporting others when they are moving through change.

Review the curve in Figure 5-2 and think about changes in your life and the reactions you experienced. Do you recognize the process you went through?

Just as with the bell curve shown earlier, the change curve is a tool you can use to assess the position at which individuals and groups are at different points in your EMR implementation. Make a list of people and groups you want to assess. Think through the behaviors they are each exhibiting, and determine where you think they are on the curve. It is a good idea to do this in a small group, so you can compare notes

Figure 5-3: Identifying and Responding to Stages of Change

Stage	Behavioral Indicators	Effective Response Options
Denial	• Withdrawal • Apathy • Avoidance / Too busy • Disbelief • Business as usual stance	• Clarify what's changing and what's not • Sell the problem, not the solution • Focus on early steps • Listen to understand points of concern • Clear up rumors • Discuss the case for change • Develop awareness
Resistance	• Fear • Anger • Confusion • Depression / Anxiety • Sabotage	• Listen actively and validate concerns • Provide information on case for change, vision and plans • Get resistors involved • Acknowledge loss • Provide support and encourage open discussion, dissent • Ensure visible sponsorship
Exploration	• Want to know more • Curious • Raising questions • Learning • Bargaining	• Ask for input / get participation • Reinforce directionally correct behavior • Continue open discussion and feedback loops • Provide training • Supervisors communicate role and department level changes • Don't bargain
Acceptance	• Commitment • Relief • Excitement • Ownership • Integration	• Practice continuous improvement • Reaffirm the vision • Reinforce new behaviors and align incentives • Continue training and support • Build confidence • Confirm workflow / other changes • Measure results / report broadly • Gather lessons learned • Celebrate success

and reach agreement on where to place people or groups. Accurate assessment is important.

Remember to assess where your sponsors are in the change cycle too. Understanding where they are and how this impacts their leadership of the change is key to providing them with effective coaching and support.

Figure 5-3 describes ways to identify where people are on the curve and suggests appropriate actions you can take in response. There are a number of change curve versions available and they use different terms to describe the reactions people have to change. Some curves are more elaborate than others. For the purposes of the Identifying and Responding to Stages of Change chart in Figure 5-3, we consolidated the stages and terms into four buckets. Use the chart to plan how you will support people based on where they are. Doing this enables you to effectively manage situations that otherwise might be problematic.

MANAGING RESISTANCE

The final topic we will cover in this chapter is managing resistance. People try to avoid resistance by pretending it isn't there and hoping it will go away. This is not effective. The best way to deal with resistance is to get it out in the open. When you know what the resistance is about, you can manage it; when you don't know what it is about, you cannot deal with it effectively.

The best way to begin managing resistance is to identify those who have the most to gain with the EMR implementation and those who have the most to lose. Those who have the most to lose are likely to resist the change. If you reframe your thinking about resistance, and see it less as defiance and more as an expression of needs, you will be more effective in your response. Find out what the specific concerns are. You may have to dig to get at the real issues.

Resistance to change is a natural and inevitable human reaction, even when the changes are self-imposed and considered positive. Remember when you decided to get married, or have a baby, or move to a new home? Did you experience regrets of any kind—buyer's remorse, cold feet? Did you even wonder what you were thinking when you made that decision? That is resistance talking. And the examples here are generally considered to be positive changes! Think about what happens when the change confronting you is externally imposed; you have no choice, and it sounds like a very bad idea.

Resistance is emotional. That is why logical arguments about why one should embrace the change don't work. The more disruptive the change, the more resistance you will see. People are most resistant when they like or are reasonably comfortable with the way things are and see the change as personally threatening.

Believe it or not, resisters play an important role in an EMR implementation. They often express what others are thinking but not saying, and this gets the issues on the table. For this reason, it is important to listen to resisters; sometimes you learn something of great importance to the project. As irritating as they can be, resisters are not necessarily illogical. Sometimes they see something that has been missed. Give resisters the opportunity to express their concerns and needs. Make it safe to question and disagree. Manage resistance by listening actively and acknowledging the concerns. This doesn't mean you have to agree with them, but you do need to listen.

Ignore resisters at your peril! Convert them to advocates by getting them involved in forming solutions. They will be very vocal supporters if they get their issues resolved and change their mind about the project.

Here is an idea for surfacing resistance:

 Exercise

Get a group together that includes resisters. Hold a discussion of concerns and, as the issues are raised, note them on a flip chart. When the list is complete, go through a process to prioritize the concerns. Assign small teams to work on the top few items. This surfaces resistance and gets the resisters involved in problem solving, giving them a sense of control and an opportunity to influence.

RECOGNIZING THE DIFFERENCE BETWEEN POSITIVE AND NEGATIVE RESISTANCE

Positive resistance is the process of exploring and testing the proposed change to gain the knowledge required to embrace the change. The questions and concerns are legitimate and lead to understanding and acceptance.

The intent of negative resistance is to derail the change. It can be active, such as lobbying others to not support the change, spreading rumors, not attending meetings, sabotaging the change effort in some way, being disruptive and refusing to participate. Less obvious signs are being "too busy" to participate, pretending to not understand organizational intent, and continually raising concerns about budget, staffing, etc.

A final word about resistance: Don't focus too much energy on resisters. Some of them may need to just go away. Let them. It is a shame when a small group of resisters succeeds in getting all the attention and sapping the energy from the project team. Your best bet is to treat resisters with respect, listen to them, and get them involved. Then focus the majority of your efforts on the people who want to succeed and just need some help to get there.

STAKEHOLDER CHECKLIST

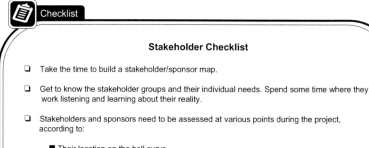

Checklist

Stakeholder Checklist

❏ Take the time to build a stakeholder/sponsor map.

❏ Get to know the stakeholder groups and their individual needs. Spend some time where they work listening and learning about their reality.

❏ Stakeholders and sponsors need to be assessed at various points during the project, according to:

- Their location on the bell curve
- Their location on the change curve
- The degree of impact they are facing
- What they stand to gain or lose with the implementation
- What they must do differently to succeed
- Level of resistance and the fundamental reason for it
- How they can best contribute to the implementation effort

❏ Develop strategies to support people/groups in moving forward based on the data gathered from this checklist.

❏ Identify and actively manage resistance. Get it out in the open.

CHAPTER 6

Communication

"Think like a wise man, but communicate in the language of the people."
– William Butler Yeats

At the highest level, the purpose of EMR project communication is to drive behavior change. Communication is successful when the desired behavior change occurs. This makes the communication function extremely important. Well-done, organized, systematic, targeted communication is the means by which most project stakeholders find out what they need to know about the EMR implementation and what is expected of them in the process.

But the behavior change that communication is driving for doesn't happen in a vacuum. In the preface to this book, we stressed the importance of recognizing the integrative nature of all the people-focused components of the project. We can't emphasize this enough. For communication to succeed, it must be received within a supportive environment that has clear sponsorship and be complemented by effective training and strengthened by a well-designed reinforcement program. This doesn't happen by itself. It requires a coordinated effort with all people-focused functions working together to align and synchronize their messages and activities.

COMMUNICATION DEFINED

Communication is more than just providing information; great communication efforts build in feedback loops to enable two-way communication in which dialog and face-to-face interactions are particularly important. Feedback is a valuable asset that helps keep the project team and sponsors in touch with stakeholder communities, gives early warning of potential issues, and is a way of surfacing resistance. It is also a key strategy in stakeholder engagement and management. By definition, interactive communication requires an interactive communication plan.

The process of pushing out information is proactive; responding to feedback is reactive. You need both. In our view, you can't have good change management without solid two-way communication!

Communication starts with stakeholder/audience identification (see Chapter 5, Stakeholder Management). The next steps are to understand how and to what degree each audience will be impacted and discover the most effective means to deliver what they need to know. You also need to understand the audience frame of reference and recognize their specific communication needs at any point. Armed with this knowledge, the communication team is positioned to:

- Be clear about the purpose of each piece of communication with each group.
- Provide the right information at the right time through a variety of channels that are relevant to specific audiences.
- Receive and respond to the feedback, which informs ongoing efforts.

This cycle repeats over and over during the course of the project. It is a process, not a set of materials. Communication is designed to impart knowledge or generate action. The process of delivering the products and receiving feedback is the means by which the purpose of communication is fulfilled. This makes the plan iterative.

The four general reasons to communicate are to:

- Raise **AWARENESS**—Provide high-level, general information about the change project; this is "for your information" type of communication.
- Develop **UNDERSTANDING**—Provide broader context and rationale for the change and give more details.
- Gain **COMMITMENT**—Get people engaged and involved, willing to take action.
- Initiate **ACTION**—Ask people to do something; ask for behavior change.

Different stakeholder groups require different types of communication at different points in the project. Some will never need more than general awareness communication. At the other end are stakeholders who need to start with awareness and move through all levels of communication to behavior change. Knowing when to apply each requires that you know and understand your stakeholder groups and the role they play in EMR implementation and technology adoption.

In this chapter, we will explore important aspects of effective communication. This is not meant to be a course on communication but rather a discussion of what we have learned (mostly the hard way!) about effective communication during large software implementation projects.

THE IMPORTANCE OF COMMUNICATION

In many ways, communication is the life blood of the project. It flows across all boundaries, impacts all stakeholders, and helps establish and maintain the tone of the project. Through communication, people learn about everything, from their first exposure to the case for change and the vision—to specific local details and the call to action, such as:

- When are we scheduled for training?
- What is our go-live date?
- What kind of on-the-ground support will we have?
- Will the new system be easier to use than what we do now?
- How will my job change?
- What is expected of me?

Good communication dispels rumors, builds confidence, and helps people feel part of what is going on. It can add a touch of humor to relieve anxiety. And when it is really good, it is a way for the organization to say to impacted employees:

> "We know you and care about you. We understand your concerns and are working to address them. We want your ideas. You are a valuable asset to the organization, and we are investing in your success. We can't do this without you—your active participation is vital."

Of course these messages must be backed up with appropriate action, but the process of communicating these things helps create an environment of trust. This is a very important contribution to the project and the organization. Great communicators who can craft these messages in a way that engages and motivates are worth their weight in gold!

"In times of change, trust-building behaviors are positively related to an organization's capacity for change. Conversely, trust-breaking behaviors are associated with a decrease in capacity for change." Margaret M. Rudolph, PhD, Consultant, Vancouver, British Columbia, Canada.

We never work on large-scale change projects without being linked at the elbow with a great communication team. Best of all, this partnership is fun—most communicators are creative and have excellent ideas about how to effectively engage people. With an implementation as significant as an EMR, we recommend you fully utilize the talents of your communication staff. Assign the best; dedicate them to the EMR effort; give them some creative license and a budget—and watch what happens. You will be amazed at what is possible.

 Key Point

Most people are very uncomfortable when they feel consciously incompetent, but care givers are particularly resistant to situations that undermine their confidence and put them into a "novice" state. There is good reason for this. A patient can be harmed by an incompetent provider. Effective communication acknowledges this concern and helps people understand how the organization will support them through the transition to competent use of an EMR.

COMMUNICATION PLANNING

You must develop a communication plan, no matter how small your organization. A communication plan can be very simple or long and complicated. What you need depends on the size and complexity of your organization.

The purpose of a communication plan is to enable delivery of planned, consistent, targeted, timely communication to the right groups, at the right times, using the most effective medium, with built-in means for two-way communication. Thinking all this through in advance improves the likelihood that your communication activities will proceed smoothly and be effective and has the added advantage of making it much easier to respond effectively to unforeseen communication needs when they arise (and they will!).

Develop the communication plan early in the project. You won't know everything at that time; just plan for what you do know, and realize that the plan will change and evolve over the course of the project, requiring regular updates.

Here are the basic things to include in a communication plan, followed by Table 6-1, which provides an example:

- Target audience/stakeholder groups.
- Objective of each communication (awareness, call to action, informational, set expectations, develop commitment, etc.).
- Vehicles/mediums for delivery.
- Who the communication is from and who is responsible for preparing it.
- Frequency and duration of the communication, if ongoing.
- Dates/Timeline for delivery.
- Feedback mechanisms.
- Status and any notes.

Table 6-1: Sample Communication Plan Template

Stakeholder Group / Person	Purpose of Communication	Vehicle / Delivery Method	Sender / Developer	Frequency / Duration	Dates / Timeline	Feedback	Status / Notes
Medical Assts.	Supporting Physicians with In Basket	Policy Revision	Labor Steward	Weekly	T-9 until Go-live	Q&A in Team Meetings	Introduce in Team Meeting

SUCCESSFUL PRACTICES
FOR EFFECTIVE COMMUNICATION

What follows are some simple truths about communicating. This is not rocket science! Much of it is common sense: Treat people with dignity and respect; tell them what they need to know—what the organization expects of them and how they will be supported. And do it in a friendly and engaging manner, using vehicles that are effective for the users.

1. Know Your People

This is the first rule. If you don't take the time to identify and understand your stakeholders, your communication efforts will not be targeted. They will be too general to be meaningful and appealing and will most likely be ignored.

Who are the stakeholders? They are all the groups, teams, committees, and individuals that have a stake in the change. Having a stake simply means that people will be impacted by the change and its outcome in some way and/or that you need something from them in order for the change to succeed.

In Chapter 5 on Stakeholder Management, we stressed the need to understand a stakeholder group's frame of reference. This means understanding the point of view, culture, language, way things are done, and the issues of the group. Another way to think of this is the WIIFM, or "What's in it for me?" This is a very important question for any individual or group. Each person wants to know what the proposed change means to him or her, good and bad. To communicate effectively, you must be able to articulate the WIIFM in the language used by the group.

Key Point

Communication Keys

Three keys to effective communication with any stakeholder group are understanding and adapting messages to their:

1. **Language** (way they speak, words they use, may mean actual language such as Spanish)

2. **Frame of Reference** (where they're coming from)

3. **What's In It For Me?**

 Quote

"One of the best ways to persuade others is with your ears – by listening to them."

- Dean Rusk

A word of advice: Get out, listen and observe how people who will be impacted by the change currently do their work. There is no substitute for this! You cannot sit in an administrative building and really understand the day-to-day reality, the issues and stressors, the workflows and the opportunities that present themselves to front-line care givers, pharmacists, receptionists, billing staff, and the many others who are impacted by an EMR implementation, unless you spend some time in their world. You can't communicate effectively if you don't know the audience—where they are coming from and the degree of impact they will experience from the change. Understanding your stakeholders enables you to make your communication style and content appropriate and effective for the intended audiences, which is the whole point.

Key Point

> To make your communication even more effective, find ways
> to help people translate EMR project messages into their own
> words. The easier it is for front-line staff to tell the story their
> way, the more likely it is that they will accept it and tell others
> about it.

Please refer to Chapter 5 on Stakeholder Management to learn more about identifying, engaging, and managing stakeholders.

2. Tell the Truth!

Be open and honest. People can smell a rat, and it's amazing how quickly this happens. In the long run, it is much easier to be honest and transparent, even about the hard issues. Here are some guidelines:

- If you don't know the answer to a question, say you don't know and then explain what you are doing to get the answer and when you expect to have it.
- Set up a regular communication schedule, so people know when they will hear from you. This reduces anxiety because people know when they will be updated and can ask questions.
  - Example: Project updates will be provided every Tuesday morning by broadcast e-mail. Q&A sessions to be held monthly by video conference. Once a quarter, all-hands lunches with leaders will be scheduled at staggered times.
- If you have a leadership role, get out and talk to the various stakeholders. Do more asking and listening than telling. Follow up on concerns that are identified. This builds trust and makes people feel valued.
- Cover both the advantages (upside) the new system will provide, and be open about anticipated issues and challenges (downside). Challenges can include anticipated difficulties with the system itself, the implementation process, or learning certain application features. This is key to managing expectations. Tell the full story. Do not sugarcoat.

- Admit when you or the project makes some kind of mistake. Believe us when we say there is no way you will get everything right on an EMR implementation! Be honest about it. Admit what went wrong; explain what's being done to fix it and how you will avoid repeating the problem.
- Acknowledge issues with past change efforts in the organization. Help people understand how these important lessons have been factored into EMR planning so they are not repeated.
- Communicate even when you don't have anything new to report. Simply state there are no changes since the last update, and things are proceeding as planned. Remind people when they can expect to hear from you again.
- In the effort to develop support for the EMR project, we stress all the advantages of the new system and talk about the problems associated with the current state. But to those who are unconvinced, this may not be believable. Counter this situation by also being candid about the potential difficulties with the EMR implementation, and acknowledge the perceived strengths of the current way of doing things. In as legitimate a way as possible, associate positive things about the current state that people want to retain to the future state described in the vision.

 Quote

"A person who has had a bull by the tail once has learned 60 or 70 times as much as a person who hasn't."

- Mark Twain

3. Gather User Lessons Learned for Continuous Improvement

One of the important things to realize about an EMR implementation is that it never really ends! After go-live, there will always be software upgrades, new applications, bug fixes, new hardware and devices, and new employees, not to mention continuing discovery of ways to improve workflow and care delivery from untapped capabilities of the system. For example, have you taken training in Microsoft Word after having used it for ten years and discovered all kinds of features and tricks you didn't know about and could have been using? That's the way EMRs are, too. It will be a continuing learning and discovery process that will translate into improved care delivery and administrative processes.

Bake the idea of continuous improvement into the project from the beginning. Help people see that everyone has a responsibility to continue learning, both from successes and mistakes. Remember, you won't get it all right the first time. Creating a continuous learning environment, "test and learn," is a strategy for dealing with this reality.

One way to introduce and reinforce the idea of continuous improvement is to gather user lessons learned after key application go-lives. This process asks users to comment on various aspects of their preparation and go-live experience to determine relative effectiveness and gather suggestions for improvement. The general areas to assess include sponsorship, communication, training, the go-live process, and support functions. We recommend conducting the inquiry six to eight weeks post go-live. This timeframe seems to be the sweet spot. Users are far enough past go-live to have stabilized, but the memory of their preparation and go-live experience is still clear.

Conducting a formal user lessons learned process helps people see that the organization is serious about improving and underscores the value of user input. It also helps to create an environment in which it is safe to try new things. When you encourage people to try things and provide opportunities for practice, they learn faster.

If your organization is large or if you are using a phased implementation approach, user lessons learned can add value immediately. A serious continuous learning message is delivered when the successes and mistakes of one go-live are used to improve the next. In fact, even users who go through a difficult go-live feel good when they know that their experience is being used to make things better for others. For this reason, we strongly recommend that you circle back to lessons learned participants to let them know how their feedback is being used to improve the project. Everyone appreciates knowing when their contribution makes a difference.

If your organization is small or if you are doing a big bang go-live, a user lessons learned process is still worth the time and effort. Gathering feedback gives users a chance to participate and be heard, and the lessons will be valuable in planning your next implementation project.

You can gather lessons learned in variety of ways—focus groups, interviews, or surveys. Whatever your method, or combination of methods, communicate the findings broadly for the biggest impact. The whole point is to share the learnings and make the identified improvements. Do this and you will be on the road to establishing a continuous learning culture.

4. Use a Variety of Mediums

You may think this goes without saying, but this rule is so important that it must be mentioned. Different communication vehicles are more effective than others with different groups. Your job is to know what methods work with your various stakeholders.

One size doesn't fit all. It's so easy to think that e-mail is the best communication method—everyone has it, it's inexpensive, and it's 24/7. What's not to like? The real question is whether e-mail is an effective vehicle for the people you are trying to reach. In some organizations, there are people who do not have computers. If you rely heavily on e-mail, they won't get the messages. And even if you are targeting managers who do have computers, it is likely that they are overwhelmed by e-mail. How will you get their attention?

The answer is that you need many different ways to reach people. E-mail is only one tool. There are many other means at your disposal: newsletters, bulletin boards, videos, CDs, conferences, meetings, broadcast voice mails, flyers, letters mailed to homes, Web sites, training programs and materials, posters, drawings and contests, demonstrations, staff meetings, supervisors, sponsors, lunches, parties and so on. Identify what currently works for your audiences and add to this with new ideas.

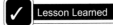

> **Lesson Learned**
>
> Spending time up front on face-to-face communication and dialog takes time, but it pays off in the long run by answering concerns, dealing directly with resistance, increasing understanding and building acceptance. Starting this early accelerates change throughout the project.

Be creative. Try new things. And measure their effectiveness. Are the communication pieces accomplishing what they are designed to accomplish? How do you know? As you identify what is most effective, do more of the things that really work. And don't forget about the people who are hard to reach. You may need to be your most creative to reach them. They will appreciate the effort.

Remember that people learn in different ways. Be sure your delivery methods include all forms—written, oral, visual, and experiential. It doesn't hurt to ask people what method of communication they prefer.

One final thought. Be mindful of when to use a formal tone and process and when to be more informal and engaging. To some extent, this is determined by the target audience. It is also influenced by whether the message content is about non-negotiables, such as legal or financial requirements, or whether you are seeking commitment to changes that are not required by law.

5. There Is No Such Thing as Overcommunicating!

People have a hard time believing that you cannot overcommunicate. In fact, the most common communication error in software deployments is under-communicating.

Has a leader ever told you that he or she has already issued the message too many times? That they feel awkward saying it again? That they believe no one wants to hear it one more time?

And yet the truth is that even if the message has been delivered multiple times, you do need to say it again. Perhaps not in exactly the same way, but you need to recommunicate the key points over and over during the life of the project. Of course you want to ensure that the message is being understood by the target audiences. If it isn't, refine it before repeating it, but keep repeating it.

Repetition and redundancy are goals, not things to be avoided. People need to hear messages multiple times before they really incorporate the meaning. Sometimes people don't fully understand what was said the first few times, or they don't believe it. The fourth or fifth time around may be when they begin to get it. This is one reason why having different communication vehicles at your disposal is so important.

There is an old saying that when the last employee *gets it,* you can stop delivering the message. This is just a fact of life. Keep communicating!

COMMUNICATION
IMPLEMENTATION CHECKLIST

❑ The purpose of communication is to drive behavior change!

❑ Build a communication plan early in the project.

❑ Ensure that early communication about the EMR implementation comes from senior leadership and clearly conveys their authorization and support.

❑ Provide scripts and talking points for leaders to help ensure consistency of messages.

❑ Clarity is a gift! Spread it around.

❑ Know your stakeholders; understand their frame of reference and what's in it for them to make the change to an EMR.

❑ Remember the need to connect with people on an emotional level.

❑ Be honest and transparent in your communication.

❑ Use communication to help manage expectations.

❑ Encourage open discussion of rumors. Failed change projects often have inaccurate rumors about the change that were not addressed.

❑ Remind people of what will stay the same.

❑ Use a variety of communication mediums and be creative in your messaging.

❑ Conduct a robust user lessons learned effort.

❑ Every communication product should have a feedback loop.

❑ Remember that avoiding pain is a greater motivator than doing something for positive reasons.

❏ For communication to succeed, it must be received within a supportive environment that has clear sponsorship and be complimented by effective training and strengthened by a well-designed reinforcement program.

❏ Communicate, communicate, communicate!

Ability—
Developing Requisite Skill

CHAPTER 7

Training Strategy

Effective training teaches people how to do their job,
not how to use the system.

An argument was made earlier about the importance of organizational context when delivering training. Training is a crucial step in the implementation process, and to be most effective, it must be delivered in an environment that supports growth and learning, and where users understand the role they play in achieving the EMR vision.

Assuming the proper context is in place, the onus is on training to "connect the dots" for users—that is, to link what users need to know with the knowledge of how and when to apply their new skills to take advantage of system capabilities. Connecting the dots is a powerful way to embed use of the system into user roles and responsibilities. It's a bigger picture way of thinking. The goal is not just to teach system features and functions but rather to support users in becoming critical thinkers who efficiently and effectively reap the benefits of the new technology.

 Key Tip

> An effective EMR user training program is user-centric meaning it is role and workflow based, not system based.

USER TRAINING DEFINED

Training is the means by which an organization teaches employees effective use of the new EMR system and consequent role changes. In other words, how does the EMR system integrate into and change the way work is done, and, as expressed in the questions that follow, what does that mean for individual roles and responsibilities? "What do I need to do differently to be successful? If I change, how will it benefit my patients and the organization?" Even the best system won't produce anticipated results if it is deployed in an environment focused on "this is how we've always done it."

Training comes in many formats—classroom, instructor-led, proctored free time, Web-based, written, etc. The best training is that which uses a combination of methods, taking into account the variety of ways adults learn. An effective EMR user training program is user-centric, meaning that it is role and workflow based, not system based. Effective training teaches people how to do their job, not how to use the system.

Here is a real-life example, as shared by a check-in clerk at one particular facility: "I attended seven hours of training, but when I got back to my desk, I didn't know how to check in a patient." This chapter presents a program called *The Connect-the-Dots Approach* that will help you avoid making this costly mistake.

THE CONNECT-THE-DOTS APPROACH

There is a rather simple way to help users connect the dots during training. The model featured in Figure 7-1 makes training relevant to users, facilitates sustainable performance improvement, and sets the stage for effective use of the newly learned computer skills on the job, creating the opportunity for meaningful use. This is done by directly connecting business reasons for the change, expectations of users, and impacts of system misuse with workflows, system training, and time for practice. There are two aspects of this: organizational and individual.

If you are successful in building relevance for users and are able to help them connect the dots, you will unleash a world of human potential other healthcare organizations will envy. It's an amazing transformation, when done well.

Figure 7-1: The Connect-the-Dots Model

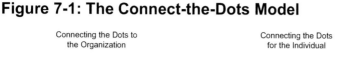

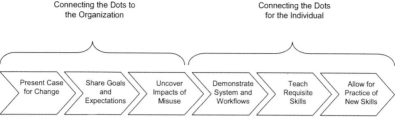

Effective training is a partnership between training and operations. Connecting the dots runs counter to transactional training approaches in which the focus is on completing feature/function training and checking it off the list. Not all training is delivered in this system-centric way, but it is not uncommon to hear complaints that training lacks a strong connection to operations. When training focuses too heavily on system features and functions, the critical clinical and business aspects are shortchanged and the real purpose is lost. This reinforces the suggestion made in Chapter 4 on the Organizational Readiness Team to involve operational thought partners in the planning process to ensure the training accurately and effectively supports operations. If operations is at the table to review, comment on and approve the training curriculum, users are sure to receive relevant role-based training. Physicians, department managers/supervisors, and labor representatives are extremely helpful partners in making certain the training content is on target.

The Connect-the-Dots Approach is a means to strengthen the relationship between training and operations by creating a partnership. When everyone agrees that training is the logical place to connect the new system with day-to-day clinical and business practice, curriculums are developed that are meaningful to users in their respective roles, scope of practice, priorities, and specialty or department. The goal is to tie the learning to a compelling case for change and to deliver the content in a way that is most useful for each audience.

Lesson Learned

It is helpful to have at least one trainer with clinical experience present when training clinical users. In the inpatient setting, using nurses as trainers can be very beneficial. Bring in retired nurses if necessary and train them well. Respected nurses can support and coach physicians in effective use of the system, helping them become productive users more quickly.

Effective training is workflow based. If you want users to understand how the technology can increase operational efficiencies, give them workflow-based training.

We recommend revising workflows as much as possible before training. But remember, you will learn a lot more about the system when you begin to use it in daily operations. That means that workflows will typically be revised more than once. Manage expectations about this. Though it may seem frustrating, revising workflows based on team experience is a great way to get people involved in leveraging the system and taking the waste out. To quote one executive, "You won't finish revising workflows until after go-live because no one knows what the damn thing (system) is before they use it in real life!"

The problem is that in a typical situation, during the scramble to prepare for implementation, trainers are not always kept abreast of clinical workflow modifications. The result is that trainers train what they know and users primarily learn features and functions of the system. Trainers demonstrate the system's capabilities but are unable to show users how the system fits into the new workflows. This may well be one of the biggest mistakes with training during an implementation, and it is usually out of the trainer's control. If workflows are not revised in time and if code is not frozen, trainers cannot build workflow-based curriculum in the production environment. It's that simple.

This is one important reason why we insist that the organizational readiness workplan be integrated with the technical workplan. Missed-opportunity situations like this must be anticipated and planned for if the organization is to get the highest value from the expensive training required for effective implementation readiness.

Key Tip

Left to their own devices, end users do **NOT** eventually figure it out over time.

Training and support are required for success. During the last few years, the notion developed that users do not need much attention and support in preparation for EMR implementations. Instead, the belief is that users will figure things out for themselves over time. This would be nice if it were true, but unfortunately it is not how things happen for most users. Technically skilled early adopters can be relatively self-sufficient, but the majority of users come from a different frame of reference, set of experiences, level of comfort with technology and other individual differences that make it difficult or impossible for them to learn on their own. The notion that users can become proficient without intervention runs counter to our experience.

Out of necessity, users do whatever they can to survive and get through their day. When they are not well prepared for change, they regress to old habits and workarounds and invent new workarounds to fill the gap. Poor preparation and attention to the people side of an implementation lead to cementing of poor workflows and inadequate use or misuse of the EMR system. There is a sense of security in use of established processes, regardless of their effectiveness. Leadership is required to ensure that new workflows are implemented and used. This doesn't happen by itself.

Over time, users may refine their abilities to use the new technology and even become better prepared to ask more sophisticated questions during follow-up training, but this is a big risk to take when so much is on the line for the healthcare organization. Given that users ultimately determine whether the EMR will deliver the hoped-for benefits, it is prudent and logical to invest in fully preparing them, pre and post go-live, to deliver results. Post-live support is essential to ensuring adoption does not stop below necessary proficiency levels, let alone the desired levels. Work after go-live is just as important as that before go-live if the changes that can be driven by technology don't fall short of potential.

Figure 7-2: Connect-the-Dots Model (Organizational Connection)

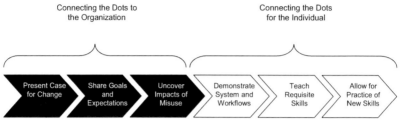

All training should build relevance from both an organizational and individual level for the users. As the training curriculum is being developed, we recommend following the Connect-the-Dots format to ensure users are engaged in their learning and get the utmost value from it.

Connecting the Dots to the Organization

Set the context for training in the beginning of a session so participants understand why they are there. Find a brief, succinct way to present the case for change, expectations of users, and how inefficient use of the system has a negative impact on the organization (see Figure 7-2). The best case scenario is to have an executive sponsor of the EMR project present this section of the training. It takes only 10-15 minutes, but the impact is incredibly powerful. Having an executive sponsor deliver this message eliminates any ambiguity about the importance of the training or the EMR implementation.

It is truly amazing to witness the dedication of some leaders as they dart from medical center to medical center (or hospital to hospital) to be present for a rolling schedule of training sessions across an organization. These individuals take the role of executive sponsor seriously and deliver the case for change in a compelling way. Making the effort to be present at initial training sessions sends a clear message and helps users see that leadership is not just paying lip service to the implementation but actually changing their behavior to champion the cause. This is an example of executive sponsorship at its best!

It is helpful to sponsors if you provide them with a script for these presentations. Review Table 7-1 for some talking point ideas. Keep in

Table 7-1: User Training Talking Points for Sponsors

Topic	Detail
Defining the business case for change	The purpose is to define what the organization is trying to accomplish via the new EMR system. Many times, the technology affords a way to improve upon a current outcome, so the executive is encouraged to compare how the organization is currently performing with how the new technology can help reach the envisioned future state.
Sharing goals and expectations from leadership	The intent is to highlight specific goals that the organization wants to accomplish and share what leadership expects of users in reaching these objectives. Share recent policy and other changes that are relevant to the discussion.
Highlighting targeted impacts	Executives help connect the dots by sharing how users directly impact patient safety, revenue capture, operational efficiencies, cost cutting, patient satisfaction, care delivery, and a host of other critical organizational priorities. Users need to understand how effective and ineffective use of EMR impacts the organization's ability to succeed. Don't assume that users are always aware that a simple click can have a major downstream impact on the patient and the organization.

mind that the message is much more believable when sponsors put it in their own words and speak with conviction. If the message is delivered by reading from a piece of paper, what gets communicated is the **lack** of passion about the topic. Users are easily turned off by this type of delivery, so coach your sponsors on how to deliver an effective message.

Figure 7-3: Connect-the-Dots Model (Individual Connection)

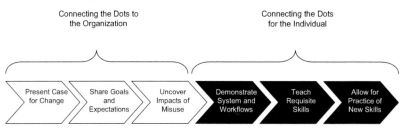

Connecting the Dots to the Organization — Connecting the Dots for the Individual

Present Case for Change → Share Goals and Expectations → Uncover Impacts of Misuse → Demonstrate System and Workflows → Teach Requisite Skills → Allow for Practice of New Skills

Connecting the Dots at the Individual Level

Connecting the dots at the individual level (see Figure 7-3) is pretty straightforward, but it is important to reiterate that the effort is greatly enhanced when the business case for change is already understood. What people need to know now is how the EMR will impact their day-to-day work and their job. Effective training delivers the answers in a way that is relevant and understandable to users. One of the best techniques is to emphasize how certain workflows and skills will benefit the user.

Physician Perspective

For the majority of physicians, technology that assists them in being both knowledgeable and efficient is quickly incorporated, whereas EMR procedures that have no immediate clinical benefit are simply felt to be a nuisance. For example, showing a provider how to bring up a list of key clinical resources with one click, while still in the patient's EMR, has been much easier to adopt than entering past surgical history, organized by CPT code, into a remote EMR entry field.

Kenneth Goodman, MD
Associate Director, Center for Continuing Medical Education
Department of Family Medicine
Cleveland Clinic

Role of front-line supervisors: It is extremely helpful to have a front-line leader (such as a clinical supervisor, physician lead, or some equivalent to a department administrator) working with the trainer in the training session. As the trainer demonstrates the new system, discusses workflows, and reviews critical new skills, users think of many questions that are beyond the ability of the trainers to answer. Instead of leaving the questions unanswered and users feeling anxious, the attending front-line leader is there to reinforce new workflows, explain role and responsibility changes, review policy adjustments, and address scope of practice concerns.

There is no better person to address these questions on the spot than a user's direct supervisor. This doesn't mean everything can be resolved in training. It does mean that users can raise their questions and get their minds back on training. The better prepared supervisors are to actively participate and support their staff, the better training and go-live will be.

Workflow: Remember that trainers should not be the first source of new information about role and other job changes. This is not their responsibility. However, trainers should be prepared to discuss workflow changes necessitated by the system, as this is critical to user ability to begin to align the system with their everyday work. Users need to clearly see the relationship between the new system and how the work of the unit gets done. The system will not be used in a vacuum but within the context of the daily activities of the unit or department. It is not good practice to allow trainers to focus on system features and functions and send users back to direct supervisors to discuss workflow related questions after training.

Remember to include discussion on how users interact with any existing systems that will stay in place and cover handoffs with ancillary departments.

Practice: Users must have adequate time to practice with the new system before going live. New skills must be ingrained. And users who are new to computers will fare much better if they can become comfortable with the computer. Build a practice environment (sandbox), and make it easy for people to access it. Ensure the sandbox mirrors the production environment and provides role and domain-specific scenarios.

Some organizations mandate practice and provide protected time for it. Some provide a practice classroom with a proctor where users practice on their own, but the proctor is available to answer questions. Supervisors must ensure everyone does practice and that questions are addressed. It is helpful if some informal leaders begin practice first and then encourage and support others to do so. Fear is a barrier to retention. Practice builds confidence.

An important aspect of effective practice is having real-life scenarios to work with. Role and specialty-specific situations help people learn how to do their real work. Ensure that the scenarios you provide are relevant to users. No hypertensive patients for surgeons!

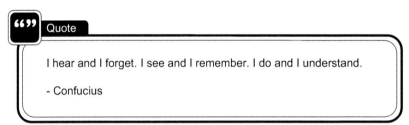

I hear and I forget. I see and I remember. I do and I understand.

- Confucius

Ancillary support: At certain points during training, it is a very helpful to have knowledgeable ancillary sponsors present, so that flow, interface, and handoff issues with orders and results can be discussed.

Updating information: We advise that you limit the number of job aids you provide. They can be overwhelming and cause confusion if not done well. To avoid the "drinking from a fire hose" syndrome, we recommend preparing a short, simple reference booklet. If you teach to the tools in the reference booklet as part of training, the tools will be used on the job.

As lessons learned are gathered, workflows are revised, and decisions are made after go-live, be sure to update the booklet and distribute to all. Have clear accountability and a process for doing this. Common complaints post-live are that changes and fixes are not consistent or are not broadly communicated. (See Table 7-2 for training principles.)

SUPPORT STRATEGY

Training is required to ensure users understand how to do their jobs effectively, but users also need on-the-ground support and continued reinforcement once the system is implemented. This is another example of the need for organizational readiness integration in which

Table 7-2: Three Guiding Principles for Effective Training

Principle	Detail
Demonstrate relevant **workflows** in new EMR system	Demonstrations of the new EMR system should be succinct and rehearsed ahead of time. Compare the way things used to be done with the new way of using the EMR. Define role and responsibility changes for those in attendance. Don't fall into the trap of showing multiple ways of accomplishing the same task, as it can overwhelm users and cause confusion. Place more emphasis on workflows and how the technology can help, not just on features and functions.
Highlight critical system **skills**	During training, users must learn critical skills by role, and develop understanding of organizational priorities and goals for use of the system. The average person cannot retain dozens of different tasks and techniques when using a new system, so it is best to focus on only what the user needs to know and limit the lessons to multiple shorter sessions, as opposed to fewer longer ones. Emphasize small things that save time and result in increased operational efficiencies. Show users how the skills relate to a manageable work/life balance. After go-live, the training should dig deeper into other features and functions within the system that can further support operations.
Provide opportunities for **practicing** the new skills	Users need to see, touch, experience, and practice the new skills and workflows. Provide adequate time during training for participants to practice so the skills can be ingrained. Also establish a practice environment (or sandbox) so users can practice outside of training at their own speed to gain comfort and confidence. It is best to provide protected time for practice to help ensure users do it.

each component supports and reinforces the other to get the desired outcomes. Training alone is not sufficient to achieve objectives. Learning must be take place in a supportive environment and must be reinforced and coached. Without reinforcement and support, it doesn't matter how much you train and communicate, you are not as likely to get the results you seek.

Because organizations differ in size, budget, and scope of applications being implemented, the intent of this section will focus more on overall strategy for supporting end users and reinforcing desired behaviors, as opposed to drilling down into the details about specific support models and ratios. It goes without saying, but the more support that can be provided in the weeks after go-live, the better.

On-the-Ground Support

The hope is that every user receives excellent training and is afforded multiple opportunities to practice newfound skills before his or her team goes live with the new system. Even with the best preparation, it is difficult to remember everything learned during training, especially when there is a rather steep learning curve. Providing on-the-ground support for users during implementation is critical to the successful transition to the new way of doing things.

On-the-ground support varies from hospital to hospital, region to region, and organization to organization. Regardless of the actual support model, the end goal should always be to help "ready users" become "confident users" of the new technology. This is important, because much too often, the support strategy is too transactional. This can be counterproductive and actually turn "ready users" into "dependent users." Transactional support is well intentioned, but it is focused on demonstrating tasks without ensuring the user can perform the tasks. This is problematic in the long run and very difficult to reverse.

The biggest mistake an organization can make is to fall into the trap of adhering to a reactive mode of delivering support in which support resources are so eager to answer questions and demonstrate how to accomplish tasks in the system that users are not actually learning. This phenomenon cripples the ability to transform users into critical thinkers because they unconsciously grow reliant on seeking help when issues or questions arise, rather than being trained to think through the situation. What happens when the support resources are no longer at the elbow? The objective should be to provide timely, targeted support in a way that leaves users capable of working through the same or similar problems on their own.

Another common mistake a support team can make is to focus too heavily on the features and functions of the system and not reinforce operational workflows. This also impedes the ability of users to transition from "ready" to "confident" status because they learn only what buttons and links to click on without fully understanding the big picture. Users definitely need to learn the requisite system skills, but more importantly, they need to know why and when to perform these functions, as well as be cognizant of the downstream effects of their actions. It is not uncommon to see waves of users struggling with the EMR even years after go-live, because they haven't been supported properly. Support resources must understand the department-specific and role-based workflows and incorporate this knowledge when providing support. And they must understand that the overall purpose of support is to create self-sufficiency, not dependency.

Remember that the best support is often provided by people who have experience doing the work. Users really appreciate having an experienced peer to learn from. This is true for both clinical and business functions. Knowledge of the workflows, terminology, and roles and responsibilities is a big plus. This is one reason why local champions, super users, and supervisors can be such great support providers.

When more weight is placed on the technology than on operations, issues are bound to arise because people get stuck and are not able to move beyond the technology. It is important to remember that the EMR is merely a tool to support operations; it shouldn't drive operations.

Growing Internal Capacity

Another focus of the overall support strategy is to effectively grow internal capacity among users. That is, users must learn to sustain themselves after a certain period of time because support cannot be provided at the rich go-live level forever. It is way too expensive. By way of analogy, parents need to learn to let go of their children at some point and trust they did everything they could to develop confident, stable, independent, and capable citizens. Just as we don't see parents accompanying their children in a college classroom or in a work setting, support resources must ensure users are able to support themselves at some defined point. This point may seem trivial, but it shouldn't be taken lightly. Much too often, organizations struggle with how to meet the growing demand for support even years after go-live, as they have created a scenario in which the project support team is viewed as the first line of defense for questions or problems that arise.

The best way to increase internal capacity on a unit is to engage early adopters and local champions in becoming active in the overall support effort from the very beginning. Additionally, front-line supervisors must be actively involved because it will be their job to monitor performance and offer first-line support as part of their ongoing role. Early adopters, local champions, super users and front-line supervisors benefit from being trained early and then repeating the training with their teams. This gives these operational support resources the knowledge that enables them to intervene effectively when team members need help. The project support resources serve as an extension of the operational support effort. They coach and mentor the front-line leaders, so they can fully assume the first line of defense role after the project support resources are disbanded.

Paying It Forward

A best practice approach for preparing front-line leaders to support their teams and champion the overall implementation effort is to have them participate with teams going live before theirs. This way the leader gets first hand go-live experience and is much better prepared for their team's event. This builds user confidence because they recognize that their leader has experience and is a credible support resource for the team. Paying it forward is a great way to develop capacity in an organization.

Another way to do this is to create a support network for the front-line supervisors. Hold weekly calls throughout the rollout schedule during which front-line leaders can talk with one another about their go-live experiences and offer advice and support. Even if front-line leaders (typically the lead nurse, clinical supervisor, and/or department administrator) aren't involved in a go-live in the near future, it is extremely helpful for them to attend the weekly call to hear the issues, challenges, and lessons learned being discussed by their peers. This is invaluable data that will help front-line leaders speak confidently with their teams about what to expect.

TRAINING CHECKLIST

 Checklist

Training Checklist

❏ Chunk the training; no one is able to drink from a fire hose.

❏ Focus only on the critical skills at go-live; show tricks and tips later.

❏ Training is part of a continuous improvement process. Provide multiple learning opportunities for users before, during, and after go-live.

❏ Training is not just about features and functions; workflows and content are king.

❏ Establish a context for sustainable learning up-front; even houses need a foundation to rest on.

❏ Focus on developing critical thinkers, not robots that just push buttons and links.

❏ Understand your definition of success, and ensure you can capture data to monitor progress toward goals.

❏ Ensure training is targeted to role, scope, and specialty to make it relevant to users.

❏ Help users understand how the implementation of the system changes relationships and handoffs between departments.

❏ Provide a sandbox for practice and exploration on own time; it must mirror production and contain role- and specialty-specific scenarios! Make sure users have sufficient time to practice before going live on the unit.

❏ Partner with Operations when delivering training to reinforce new workflows/roles/responsibilities and help integrate the system into the day-to-day work.

❏ Be strategic with job aids; keep them short and simple to not overwhelm. Teach to the aids in training. Keep them updated as things change.

❏ Make sure front-line leadership/sponsors are trained ahead of time, so they know what they are preaching and can support their teams. They should play an active role in training, workflow redesign, role and responsibility changes, and issue resolution. Support them with timely information such as scripts, frequently asked questions, training schedules, go-live dates, etc.

CHAPTER 8

Reinforcement

Reward what you want to see.

Reinforcement is the most underutilized means of driving behavior change in organizations. Reinforcement is a means of making the incentive to change greater than the incentive to stay the same. Leveraging the power of reinforcement delivers clarity of purpose and focused energy to your EMR implementation and by so doing, speeds up the process of change.

REINFORCEMENT DEFINED

Reinforcement refers to all means an organization utilizes to recognize and reward desired behavior and deliver negative consequences for undesired behavior. When reinforcement aligns incentives with the desired future state, it is a key driver for achieving business objectives:

> "...in the workplace, there is no accelerator with more impact than purpose-based recognition."[4]

Please note that we use the word *reinforcement* intentionally because it encompasses both positive and negative response to employee actions.

 Key Tip

Reinforcement = Rewards + Negative Consequences

Don't dismiss reinforcement as just "soft stuff" or "being nice," sentiments often associated with appreciation programs in which rewards are not tied to clearly defined behavior changes and outcomes. Reinforcement isn't about thanking people for extra effort—the real question is not how hard someone worked but what was accomplished. There is nothing wrong with appreciating employees, but a well-designed reinforcement program is much more than appreciation.

Reinforcement programs with strategic intent require:

- Clarity about the specific behaviors and performance outcomes you are looking to reward. Employees must understand the desired target.
- Company-wide understanding that good performance against the stated expectations will be rewarded, while there will be negative consequences for poor performance.
- Expectation-setting with leaders so they understand that delivering reinforcement is part of their job. Reinforcement is a tool to help the organization stay on purpose, drive to desired outcomes, and maintain momentum.
- Reinforcement guidelines for leaders so they know the full range of reward and consequence options available, as well as the process for delivering them. To provide this, you must have a reinforcement program in place.
- Assurance that leaders are prepared to do a good job delivering both positive and negative reinforcement. Many people are uncomfortable delivering negative consequences. But don't overlook the fact that some people even feel uncomfortable delivering positive feedback. Both of these skills can be learned and developing them is a productive investment.
- Connection with emotions. Reinforcement efforts that don't evoke feelings miss the mark.

 Key Point

It's not enough to just tell people **what** outcomes are expected. People need to know **how** to achieve the outcomes. When you tie reinforcement to specific behaviors or actions, it's easy for people to understand how they can be successful.

We want to drive home two critical success factors:

1. Because actions speak louder than words, effective reinforcement programs are:
   - Predictable;
   - Consistent;
   - Specific;
   - Certain;
   - Immediate;
   - Applied fairly; and
   - Aligned with company values and objectives.
2. Employees who are prepared to succeed:
   - Are clear about what they are expected to achieve and how to get there;
   - Have the skills to meet the expectations;
   - Have the time available to achieve the expectations;
   - Know how their performance will be evaluated; and
   - Receive regular feedback on performance.

Anything less in either area causes confusion, and confusion slows down change. In other words, doing these two things well accelerates change.

THE IMPORTANCE OF REINFORCEMENT

Without reinforcement, leaders who talk about project vision and goals are just cheerleaders. It's the reinforcement program that makes organizational priorities clear and backs up words with action.

Corporate America is fond of saying "you get what you measure," but it's really "you get what you reinforce," which means you get what you pay attention to. When measurement is a means of reinforcement, it is a tool that drives behavior change. Think of reinforcement as a day-to-day management tool, not just something to be pulled out on special occasions.

 Key Tip

Don't let the perfect be the enemy of the good. Recognize progress and directionally-correct behavior in addition to success. Success is most often the cumulative effect of many small steps.

INCENTIVE ALIGNMENT

One big pitfall in change management efforts is not aligning formal incentives. We ask people to change behavior and then we continue to reward them for old behaviors. Guess which behaviors people exhibit in this situation. We can't overemphasize the need to purposefully acknowledge and reward people for the new way, not the old. Misaligned incentives can derail your project.

Ensure that your technology adoption plan includes a section for reinforcement. A critical piece of this is to work with your Human Resources team to review the performance management system. Assess the gap between what employees are currently being incentivized to deliver, compared with what they need to deliver in the new world of EMRs. What are the behaviors and outcomes you are seeking? How can the formal performance management system align with and support the objectives of the EMR implementation? Aligning strategic performance incentives with EMR objectives is a foundational building block for success.

Remember that all incentive programs for all employees impacted by the EMR implementation must be evaluated and realigned.

For example: It does no good to send front-line staff to EMR training, provide on-the-ground support for them, and incentivize them to use the new system in their daily work but forget to align the incentives of middle leadership to the EMR project. When middle leaders and their front-line staff drive to different goals, the result is confusion, morale issues, and failure to meet objectives. Don't make this costly and preventable mistake!

 Key Tip

> If your project is suffering from inconsistent sponsorship try incorporating accountability for EMR implementation success into sponsor incentive plans—and watch sponsor engagement and performance improve.

KNOW YOUR PEOPLE

Rewards and recognition have significantly more impact when they are thoughtfully targeted to individuals or groups. "Generic" acknowledgement is well-meaning but misses the real value of the emotional connection with people. It is not always possible to make every reinforcement situation personal, but it pays to take advantage of knowing your people's preferences and responding accordingly whenever possible. If you are a manger, it is your responsibility to know what is meaningful to your team members. When you make rewards personal, you communicate that people matter.

Example: If you have staff with small children, aged parents, or family members with disabilities, you probably know that flexibility with work hours is highly valued. Though these employees may appreciate being recognized and given a branded coffee mug, a tee-shirt, or a movie ticket, you might be able to have a bigger impact the next time they get a call from home by allowing them the freedom to deal with the problem without feeling conflicted. This is admittedly easier to do in administrative areas, but when possible, this attention to the employee's real needs goes a long way in building loyalty and incentive to go the extra mile for the organization when needed. Add a specific acknowledgement and thank them for great EMR-related work, as you let them leave early to handle their personal situation and you have connected the reward with project performance in their mind.

The following tool is a guide. Use it to develop greater understanding of your people to make reinforcement efforts more meaningful. You can ask people to use the form to indicate what their preferences are, you can interview them, or you can jot down ideas about individual preferences as you learn more about people in the course of working together. Either way, you are identifying rewards and recognition options that are highly valued by your people.

A word of caution: Not everyone appreciates public recognition. Making the assumption that everyone wants the spotlight is a common mistake. Getting to know your people will ensure that you offer praise and recognition in a way that feels good to the employee, ensuring the greatest positive impact.

"Perks like tuition reimbursement can never take the place of a front-line supervisor who sets clear goals, communicates, builds trust, holds employees accountable, and then recognizes in an effective manner."[4]

Tool

Rewards & Recognition Preferences

Name: _____

I prefer recognition that is:
❏ Public   ❏ Private   ❏ Either

I most appreciate receiving recognition from *(check all that apply)*:
❏ My supervisor   ❏ My team members
❏ My supervisor's boss   ❏ Anyone who thinks I have done a good job
❏ Other company leaders   ❏ Other: _____

I value being acknowledged when I *(check all that apply)*:
❏ Achieve my goals
❏ Make an extra effort, go out of my way
❏ Do something special for a patient
❏ Complete a significant project
❏ Other: _____

Rewards that are valuable to me include *(check all that apply)*:
❏ Public recognition   ❏ Bonus or other monetary reward
❏ Thank you from my supervisor   ❏ Company logo items/gear
❏ Thank you from team members   ❏ Training opportunities
❏ Team events like a lunch or dinner   ❏ Lunch with a senior executive
❏ A day off   ❏ Scheduling flexibility
❏ A preferred assignment

Additional comments about your recognition preferences:

Key Tip

Positive reinforcement has the most impact when the rewards are meaningful to users. The way to get this right is to know your people!

POSITIVE REINFORCEMENT

Rewards, recognition, incentives, and yes, even appreciation, come in many forms. Know your people, understand your company guidelines, and be creative. Combine the three and you will be on the way to unleashing the power of reinforcement to move your organization forward.

Most companies have standard guidelines in place. If you are a leader, it is your responsibility to be familiar with what the company provides. Authorized tangible and intangible rewards are important in part because they come from the top of the organization. Make sure your people understand that executive leadership approves and authorizes these rewards for your use in recognizing and rewarding their performance.

But don't take the easy way out and rely solely on the formalized reinforcement of your performance management system—performance appraisal, salary and bonus, promotion and incentive plan. Though these programs are very important means of establishing structured foundational support for rewarding employees, they are by no means exhaustive. And they are typically the least flexible of your options. Another limitation with formal programs is that they usually happen long after the fact. Reinforcement is most effective when it occurs as close to the event being acknowledged as possible.

In many cases, just beginning to use company reinforcement mechanisms as a tool to support behavior change can make a big difference. Companies budget for rewards and recognition, but these funds are not always fully utilized. Don't worry about trying to have the most creative program around at first. Simply using what is readily available may be just what you need to get started. As you focus more on knowing your people and working within your guidelines, you can expand your efforts.

If you are having trouble getting started with reinforcement, you might want to consider engaging a small group of employees to come up with reward ideas that will resonate with their peers. Ensure the team sticks to company guidelines and ask them to identify both tangible and intangible ideas, so there are a variety of choices, and not all of them require budget.

Remember, a simple, sincere thank you is sometimes all you need to give. We have heard so many stories about the handwritten thank you notes sent to employee homes being posted on the refrigerator, the thank you e-mail saved in a file for years, and the pride of receiving a public thank you. We can't recommend this simple method enough. It's easy, doesn't require planning ahead, and the price is right.

Be sure to celebrate. Even directionally-correct behavior and small successes deserve attention as you seek to build momentum. Go for some early wins and celebrate together. Social time builds relationships and teamwork.

Positive reinforcement isn't valuable only because it rewards specific efforts or outcomes but because it also is a means of reinforcing company values and objectives.

Employee Personal Responsibility

This chapter has discussed ways organizations can encourage people to make desired changes and reward them according to performance outcomes, but employees have responsibility too. Ask them to step up and learn to use the EMR effectively and contribute to a successful implementation. Committed employees do a better job. In healthy relationships, accountabilities go both ways. Be clear about what you will do for your people, and be clear about what you expect from them in return.

NEGATIVE CONSEQUENCES

Negative consequences for poor performance are usually dictated by company human resource policy. Serious options include issuing formal warnings, initiating a formal improvement plan, and at the extreme, termination. But long before you get to this point, you must deliver clear messages about your expectations, what you think it will take to turn things around, and when you must see changes.

Generally you start with a discussion of the perceived gap between what is expected and what is being delivered. Give the employee a chance to respond to your concerns. Try to reach an agreement about how performance will improve. And let the employee know what the next steps will be if the desired changes are not made. Follow company guidelines, and if you don't see results, move to the next level. If the situation is serious you should consult with your human resources representative. But don't dodge the issue!

Another way to apply negative consequences is to reduce or eliminate rewards and recognition for non-performers. This is a more subtle approach but can be very effective.

Another reinforcement method is to make old ways progressively harder to do, while simultaneously making the new way easier. The new EMR system will automatically make some processes more desirable. If you can intervene to intentionally make old ways increasingly difficult to do, you will be ahead of the game. Some examples of this include only accepting paper forms two days a week, providing short turnaround on electronic submissions with delays built into paper submissions, charging a department for continued use of transcription services, not allowing certain processes to be conducted on paper after a certain date, and so on.

 Checklist

Reinforcement Checklist

❏ EMR implementations change many things in an organization, and this is an evolving process. Help leaders effectively support staff by ensuring they understand new performance expectations and what a good job looks like with the EMR in place.

❏ Facilitate delivery of reinforcement by making it easy for leaders to understand the rewards and consequences they have at their disposal.

❏ Make sure leaders know they are accountable for providing reinforcement that supports new expectations. If they are slow to take on reinforcement responsibilities try reminding them.

❏ Help leaders understand how to use reinforcement constructively and effectively to achieve the behaviors and outcomes the organization is seeking. The more comfortable they are, the more often they will do it sincerely—and the more impact it will have.

❏ Remember that public recognition sends clear messages about what's expected and what will be rewarded. Most employees will respond to this.

❏ When employees know their contributions are valued and rewarded, they are more engaged and more accountable.

❏ Align the value of the reward with the importance of the contribution.

❏ Ask employees to commit to doing their part to ensure a successful transition to electronic medical records. The organization will do a lot for users during the implementation; employees do their part by fully engaging and contributing.

Chapter 9

Implementation Readiness

Just what the doctor ordered...

There is a great deal of activity in the months leading up to go-live to ensure the organization is well-positioned for a successful launch. With a clear focus on the people side of the implementation, much attention is centered on preparing users to effectively incorporate the EMR into daily operations.

Assuming the appropriate context is in place to reinforce and sustain desired behavior change, the objective is not only to equip users with the necessary skills and information they'll need to be effective in the transition but also to execute a strategy aimed at instilling a much needed level of confidence and critical thinking in users. Experiencing an EMR implementation can conjure up a slew of emotions and thoughts, ranging from sheer delight to anger, utter frustration, and self-doubt. The goal is to provide users with a supportive context, adequate training, and enough opportunities to build confidence so that a seamless transition into life with an electronic medical record system occurs.

Experience has shown that the faster an individual can adapt to life using the new technology well, the more likely the user will overcome the distractions inherent in an implementation and think more critically about how best to leverage the EMR system to achieve organizational goals. If users are overwhelmed with the technology and the changes inherent in the process of going live, they will continue to be distracted to the point where they remain focused on just getting through the day.

Organizations fare much better when they help users overcome their challenges before implementation because having to address these issues after go-live impedes the organization's ability to optimize, grow, and realize a return on investment. If a process is not established early on that focuses on the people side of the implementation, the organization will lose momentum and be faced with having to backtrack. This is a significant undertaking after the fact and can be extremely expensive and frustrating.

To much surprise for some executives and operational leaders, many users still struggle with the system even years after go-live. These individuals are either identified through performance indicators or fall through the cracks and go unnoticed and unsupported. Whatever the reason, a struggling user means the EMR is not being utilized effectively, which results in less than optimal outcomes for patients and the organization. Needless to say, a struggling user is also one who is literally drowning in work, as exhibited by physicians who fall behind in their InBasket or in completing their documentation. Over time, people become reluctant to seek help because it seems safer to hide under the radar, go unnoticed, and not risk the humiliation of being thought incompetent. These problems are difficult to unravel after implementation. Hopefully, by raising these concerns, we will convince you to develop a strong preimplementation people strategy.

IMPLEMENTATION READINESS DEFINED

If you ask people in the healthcare industry how they would describe a ready user, you are likely to hear a variety of definitions. Most often the criteria that surfaces centers on possessing fundamental computer skills (e.g., typing, using a mouse, surfing the Internet, managing files, copy/paste, keyboard shortcuts), acquiring the requisite EMR system feature/function skills, and having a good handle on department workflows.

The Ready User Model featured in Figure 9-1 argues that faster returns are obtained when your strategy shapes users into being better business partners and critical thinkers. Placing too much emphasis on the technology develops users who learn what buttons to click but are rarely able to explain the downstream impact of their actions. They tend to be myopically focused on just completing tasks within

Figure 9-1: Ready User Model

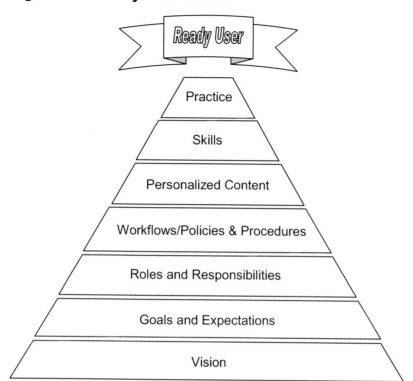

the system when the real objective in shaping ready users is to instill a deeper level of understanding of the system and its direct impact on individual, departmental, and organizational outcomes. Consider the Ready User Model shown in Figure 9-1.

The Ready User Model suggests that there is a hierarchy of needs a user must satisfy to truly become a "ready user." The idea is that individuals want to make sense of their world and they benefit from knowing how their actions and performance contributes to the bigger picture. As the context continues to build from the bottom toward the peak of the pyramid, users see greater relevance and become more engaged in the training and support they receive leading up to implementation.

The first readiness factor, **Vision,** sets the stage by defining the overall purpose of the EMR implementation and describing the desired future state. It refers to the vision of the organization and helps users see the light at the end of the tunnel. It should be compelling, exciting, and possible.

The second readiness factor, **Goals and Expectations,** is a natural extension of Vision because it brings clearer purpose to users. Both parts of the factor, goals and expectations, translate the vision into actionable targets. Goals are a step closer to reality and enable users to connect more easily with what work needs to be done. Goals and expectations are critical organizational factors in establishing a suitable context for change.

The third factor, **Roles and Responsibilities,** provides context for users because they can better see how they fit into the bigger picture. When users can make the connection between themselves and the organization, they become engaged in the preparation process. This factor is also critical in establishing a suitable context for overall change.

The fourth factor, **Workflows/Policies and Procedures,** is yet a closer look at how users fit into the change effort. Getting involved in decisions that drive internal efficiencies on the unit and how these modified processes improve the effectiveness of the team helps to further personalize the context surrounding users. Individuals see more clearly how they fit into the changes that lie ahead and how they contribute to benefits realization.

The fifth factor is **Personalized Content**. EMR systems offer sophisticated automated tools that enable users to be more efficient, effective, and faster at navigating through the technology and providing targeted care to patients. Establishing personalized content helps users configure the system in a way that is more consistent with and more supportive of their work style. As they further understand how the system can better support their daily operations, users become more fully engaged.

Physician Perspective

When it comes to physicians, it's all about saving time during the day. The key to speed is staying away from the mouse and utilizing the system tools, such as .phrases (dot phrases). Use of these tools reduces the need for much manual data input, and actually leads to two actions (data input as well as data extraction) with one stroke. This makes things faster for the physician and makes the overall decision process more sound and efficient.

Safaa Al-Haddad, MD
Internal Medicine
University Hospitals
Cleveland, Ohio

The sixth factor, **Skills,** speaks directly to attaining requisite system skills and ensuring the user is capable of appropriately completing a patient's chart and performing other key functions according to the organization's expectations. Interestingly, many people seem to think that feature/function training is the only way to bring people up to speed. The Ready User Model argues that training is more effective and sustainable when done within an appropriate context, as one step in an overall process.

The seventh and final factor, **Practice,** is incredibly important for users to really build confidence using the new EMR system. The old adage that "practice makes perfect" is right on the money. Users need ample time and opportunity to practice their skills in an environment typically known as the *sandbox,* the practice environment that mimics the final production site. During practice, users get to play around with the system without tainting real patient records, allowing them to gain needed comfort with the technology before having to use it when it counts. Without enough time for practice, users are not able to prepare adequately for go-live and, therefore, will not be good critical thinkers on the job. If users are distracted by the technology, it will interfere with their ability to treat patients. Adequate practice is essential.

When all seven readiness factors are satisfied, users can comfortably grow into ready user status. They will have the skills and the confidence to meet performance expectations. Training people is easy but developing critical thinkers and business partners who have an eye on the end goal is much more difficult, but also much more beneficial. In Chapter 7 on Training Strategy, we go into this in more detail, outlining a recommended strategic approach to the delivery of training and discussing factors that impact training effectiveness.

THE IMPLEMENTATION READINESS PROGRAM

A proven method for ensuring front-line leaders and users are well-prepared for go-live and life after go-live is to execute a planned implementation readiness program for all departments, specialties, and domains of practice. Our recommended process, the Implementation Readiness Program, occurs during the months leading up to go-live, provides support and training during go-live, and then concludes with five weeks of additional support post live. It is a defined, systematic hierarchy of steps designed to build skill, confidence and critical thinking ability.

The Implementation Readiness Program consists of four segments or stages (see Figure 9-2), which take place sequentially as described next. The entire program runs for 20 weeks, from T-14 to T+5 (referring again to Figure 9-2).

Figure 9-2: Four Stages of the Implementation Readiness Program

	Timeline	Focus	High-Level Detail
1	T-14 → T-11	Leader Implementation Readiness	Series of four weekly prep meetings for front-line leaders
2	T-10 → T-11	User Pre-Live Readiness	Series of ten weekly prep meetings for users, facilitated by front-line leaders
3	T- 0	Go-Live Team Training	Just-in-time Training
4	T+1 → T+5	User Post-Live Team Meetings	Series of five weekly meetings for teams facilitated by front-line leaders

WHO FACILITATES THE USER PRE-LIVE READINESS, GO-LIVE TEAM TRAINING, AND USER POST-LIVE TEAM MEETINGS?

The Organizational Readiness Team (ORT) plays a key role in planning and executing the implementation readiness meetings, but the best practice approach is to support the front-line leadership team in facilitating these meetings. This generally necessitates some coaching and mentoring, as many front-line leaders are not comfortable serving in this role. However, good front-line leadership results in better team performance in the long run, so it is worth the effort to prepare all front-line leaders to be effective sponsors and facilitators of their team's preparation for implementation. The Leader Implementation Readiness meetings are the first part of the Implementation Readiness Program. These sessions are designed to prepare front-line leaders for their important role in preparing teams for go-live and supporting them post-live.

1. LEADER IMPLEMENTATION READINESS

The Leader Implementation Program consists of four planning sessions, for which the ORT partners with each department or team front-line leadership group. The leadership group may consist of a physician lead, department administrator or clinical supervisor, and a union steward or lead.

As stated in Figure 9-2, there is a series of four weekly preparatory meetings for front-line leaders (see Figure 9-3), facilitated by the ORT. The objective is to prepare these leaders to effectively lead their team(s) through the User Pre-Live Readiness stage of the program (see Figure 9-4).

Figure 9-3: Stage One of the Implementation Readiness Program

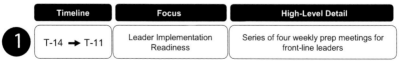

Timeline	Focus	High-Level Detail
T-14 → T-11	Leader Implementation Readiness	Series of four weekly prep meetings for front-line leaders

Figure 9-4: Leader Implementation Readiness Meetings

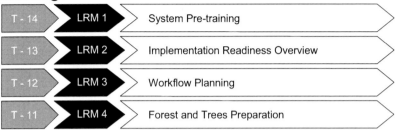

Figure 9-5: Leader Readiness Meeting #1

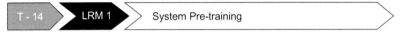

Objective

The objective of the Leader Readiness Meeting #1 (see Figure 9-5) is to ensure that all front-line leaders are trained in advance of their staff. This guarantees that the leaders are comfortable and know what to do to lead their team; and they are familiar with system capabilities, so they can better champion the technology.

Timing

Held 14 weeks before go-live (four weeks before the team Implementation Readiness Meetings begin).

Duration

Training may vary and be spread out over time. Front-line leaders should begin with a Web-based overview course and then attend instructor-led courses.

Details

Front-line leaders will repeat system training with their teams. The benefit of being pre-trained is that it gives leaders the experience to better support their teams during training. This early knowledge also prepares leaders for workflow and role redesign and any potential pol-

icy and procedure changes. Pre-training is good modeling and reinforces the importance of the EMR implementation.

Figure 9-6: Leader Readiness Meeting #2

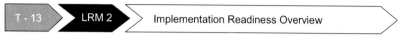

T - 13 | LRM 2 | Implementation Readiness Overview

Objectives

The objectives of the Leader Readiness Meeting #2 (see Figure 9-6) are
to provide an overview of the implementation process, reiterate the
front-line leader's role, and introduce the support resources that will
help them facilitate their teams through the preparation process.

Timing

Held 13 weeks before go-live (three weeks before the team Implementation Readiness Meetings begin).

Duration

Two to four hours.

Details

Leader Implementation Readiness Meeting #2 provides front-line
leaders with all of the information they need to understand the change
they and their teams are about to experience. Logistics are also covered. The team readiness schedule is reviewed so rooms can be booked
for these sessions.

Figure 9-7: Leadership Readiness Meeting #3

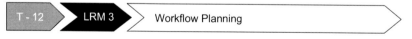

T - 12 | LRM 3 | Workflow Planning

Objectives

The objectives of the Leader Readiness Meeting #3 (see Figure 9-7) are
to review the workflows under consideration and to discuss a process
for reaching team decisions about consequent changes to roles and
responsibilities.

Timing

Held 12 weeks before go-live (two weeks before the team Implementation Readiness Meetings begin).

Duration

Four hours.

Details

Leader Implementation Readiness Meeting #3 is important because front-line leaders need to understand how workflow discussions impact the overall success of team preparation. Front-line leaders need an opportunity to review their workflows to determine which decisions can be left to the team and which decisions will be determined at a leadership level. The decisions made at a leadership level should be made prior to introducing the workflows to the team and are considered "non-negotiables." Front-line leaders introduce the workflows to the team and partner with the ORT to demonstrate the associated tasks in the EMR system.

Figure 9-8: Leadership Readiness Meeting #4

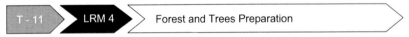

Objective

The objective of the Leader Readiness Meeting #4 (see Figure 9-8) is to ensure front-line leadership is prepared to deliver the Forest and Trees presentation (see Figure 9-12) to their teams in the upcoming team Implementation Readiness Meeting #1.

Timing

Held 11 weeks before go-live (one week before the team implementation readiness meetings begin).

Duration

Four hours.

Details

Front-line leaders are provided the Forest and Trees presentation and asked to determine who will deliver which parts. Given that each team may have two to three different leads (physician, nurse, union representative, manager), it is important to coordinate speaking parts.

Leaders are most believable and compelling when they can put the presentation into their own words. The Presentation Personalization Guide (see next "Tool" box) can help sponsors craft their own messages.

Presentation Personalization Guide

- Based on what I know, this is what I am excited about…
- What concerns me the most is…
- This is how I am preparing for our implementation…
- This is how I see using the system…
- This is how I believe we can support one another…
- I know our patients are really going to be pleased with…
- Our team in particular will benefit from this technology because…

2. USER PRE-LIVE READINESS

The User Pre-Live Readiness Program (see Figure 9-9, Stage Two) provides users with an opportunity to understand how they fit into the big picture as it equips them with the necessary skills and knowledge to be successful. Executing the program requires organizational com-

Figure 9-9: Stage Two of Implementation Readiness Program

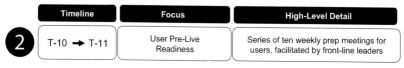

Timeline	Focus	High-Level Detail
T-10 → T-11	User Pre-Live Readiness	Series of ten weekly prep meetings for users, facilitated by front-line leaders

Figure 9-10: User Implementation Readiness Program

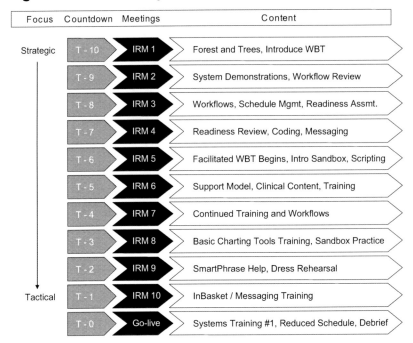

Focus	Countdown	Meetings	Content
Strategic	T - 10	IRM 1	Forest and Trees, Introduce WBT
	T - 9	IRM 2	System Demonstrations, Workflow Review
	T - 8	IRM 3	Workflows, Schedule Mgmt, Readiness Assmt.
	T - 7	IRM 4	Readiness Review, Coding, Messaging
	T - 6	IRM 5	Facilitated WBT Begins, Intro Sandbox, Scripting
	T - 5	IRM 6	Support Model, Clinical Content, Training
	T - 4	IRM 7	Continued Training and Workflows
	T - 3	IRM 8	Basic Charting Tools Training, Sandbox Practice
	T - 2	IRM 9	SmartPhrase Help, Dress Rehearsal
Tactical	T - 1	IRM 10	InBasket / Messaging Training
	T - 0	Go-live	Systems Training #1, Reduced Schedule, Debrief

mitment and relies heavily on leadership to ensure adequate time is allotted for the team to convene and work through their preparation together.

Organizations differ in size, number of locations, and so forth, so the exact implementation readiness approach will need to be customized to meet the needs of your users. The User Pre-Live Readiness program highlighted in Figure 9-10 offers a structure that is intended to develop user confidence and critical thinking, both crucial for a successful go-live and an effective transition through subsequent phases of the project life cycle. The objective is to begin with a broad picture of the future and successively drill down and connect the dots for users so they can understand their roles in meeting targets.

The User Pre-Live Readiness Program structure outlines a ten-week schedule of meetings leading up to go-live. The initial kickoff meeting is strategic in nature, and then subsequent meetings drill down into much greater detail pertaining to what users can expect at go-live. The first meeting occurs ten weeks before go-live (or T-10) and the last readiness meeting occurs one week before go-live (or T-1). Training and support continue weeks after go-live, and this will be discussed in detail after exploring the activity that takes place before implementation.

Figure 9-11: User Pre-Live Readiness Meeting #1

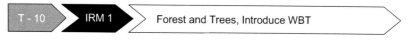

Objectives

The objectives of Implementation Readiness Meeting #1 (see Figure 9-11) are to kick off the implementation experience and provide a department or team with an overview of the EMR technology capabilities and promised benefits, what users can expect during the coming months, and an explanation of the rollout schedule.

Timing

It is suggested that this first readiness meeting take place ten weeks before go-live.

Duration

Ideally, the meetings should be two to four hours in duration. The time allotment will vary, depending on the number of participants. Provide enough time to allow for discussion.

Details

This first meeting is with a department or team as a whole. An executive sponsor should present the overall strategy and vision and describe the purpose of implementing an EMR. The goal is to paint a compelling picture of the future that engages users. Keep in mind that this may be the first time employees hear about the EMR project. Some may have been tainted by rumors about drastic changes ahead. This is a great time for the executive sponsor to connect with users and create excitement and energy around the technology and the anticipated benefits. It is also a time for users to ask questions and air concerns openly.

During this first meeting, a "Forest and Trees" presentation is delivered to engage users in the bigger picture (or forest) and drill

Figure 9-12: Forest and Trees Concept

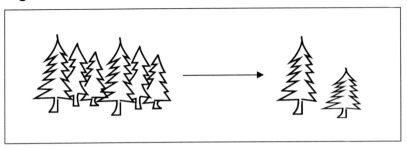

down to details that are important to them (the trees). This presentation sets the stage for implementation readiness meetings to follow. It
builds user understanding of the overall purpose and objectives of the
project and provides a high-level view of what users will experience in
the implementation process.

Just like the Forest and Trees presentation used during the first
meeting, the entire Implementation Readiness Program takes the
approach of starting broadly and then drilling down into more detail
through successive meetings until users know what they need to know
to succeed at go-live and beyond.

A good Forest and Trees overview presentation (see Figure 9-12)
communicates, but is not limited to, the following key pieces of
content:

- What an EMR is and why it is being implemented.
- The future state vision.
- How the EMR fits into the overall strategy of the organization.
- The benefits and opportunities presented by the technology (for
  patients and the organization).
- Things that might be difficult during the implementation.
- Anticipated returns on the investment.
- What will change (how things are currently, how things will be
  different).
- Project details, overview.
- Project governance structure.
- Implementation schedule (rollout plan).
- Support model (how users will be supported).
- Clinical content (what is it, why it is important).

- Sources for additional information.
- System overview, and if time allows, an opportunity to play with the system.
- Sponsor endorsement of the product and the implementation project.
- Readiness plan and logistics.

The first implementation meeting is an ideal time to ensure users clearly understand that they are expected to actively participate throughout the entire readiness process. Sponsors should strongly encourage users to take an initial pass through the Web-based training (WBT) before they attend Implementation Meeting #2 the following week. This is an important step in preparing users to contribute to workflow discussions. Users need to develop some understanding of the EMR early, so they don't become lost and therefore disengage from the process.

A powerful way to encourage users to take the WBT is to ensure that all sponsors and front-line leaders take it before the Implementation Readiness Program begins. This enables the sponsors to speak from experience and share how the WBT helped them gain an understanding of what the system is all about and how it will support operations. This is an example of sponsors modeling the behavior they expect from users.

A best practice in preparing users for upcoming workflow discussions is to provide predesigned video demonstrations (e.g., developed in Camtasia, Captivate, or some other video capture software program). Encourage users to view these videos on the organization's intranet. Users often adopt the videos faster than the WBT because the videos are generally very short in duration (between one and four minutes) and do not require any action other than watching demonstrations of a task within the system. The videos can be viewed at the user's convenience—between patients, on break, or at home (if the user has virtual access to the intranet). Sponsors should strongly encourage users to utilize both the WBT and the video demonstrations to prepare for the next Implementation Readiness Meeting. Remember, the WBT and videos are only effective if people watch them. This is enabled by ensuring everyone has access to a computer, and it helps if users have dedicated time to initiate their learning.

It is important to note that users will need to possess a fundamental level of computer skills in order to use the EMR system. This first Implementation Readiness Meeting is a good time to communicate how users can develop their computer skills and stress the importance of not waiting until go-live to address this. At ten weeks before go-live, there is still enough time to get help, practice, and fine-tune these skills. It is strongly suggested that the ORT incorporate a fundamental computer and typing skills assessment into the readiness process, as well as offer courses and support for users who may require it.

Figure 9-13: User Pre-Live Readiness Meeting #2

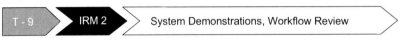

T - 9 | IRM 2 | System Demonstrations, Workflow Review

Objectives

The objectives of Implementation Readiness Meeting #2 (see Figure 9-13) are to initiate discussion around impacted workflows and to show live demonstrations of the system's capabilities as it pertains to these workflows.

Timing

Nine weeks before go-live.

Duration

Four hours in duration. Typically, there are 80+ different workflows to review with the team, and it requires a significant amount of discussion and system walkthroughs to identify points at which roles, responsibilities, tasks, and flow may change at go-live.

Details

Implementation Readiness Meeting #2 typically occurs a week after the kickoff meeting, and involves a detailed exploration of how key workflows of the team might change. Some workflow changes may be predetermined by leadership, but there are opportunities to tailor much of the flow to support how the team delivers care. When leadership predetermines certain aspects of a workflow, it generally means that the change is non-negotiable and is a result of a desire to standardize certain processes for consistency or to streamline a known pain point. Do not make the mistake of just letting the EMR automate the way the team presently delivers care. Workflows discussions are an opportune time to work as a team to find better ways of delivering care, sorting out inefficiencies and streamlining processes to transform the way care is delivered.

Part of readiness preparation involves running through relevant workflows using the system to demonstrate the system capabilities. This helps users get a sense of how the system will support them with daily operations. Workflow demonstrations need to be repeated to ensure everyone in the group is following along at a comfortable pace. The team also needs to think through any role changes that might be required to increase efficiencies when using the system. Of course, this process is always smoother when users have taken the initiative to learn about the system prior to the meeting by leveraging the WBT and video demonstrations on the Intranet.

During this meeting, it is extremely helpful for the front-line supervisor or lead physician to review organizational goals with the team and ensure the team is working productively to incorporate the impending changes into their daily operations.

Figure 9-14: User Pre-Live Readiness Meeting #3

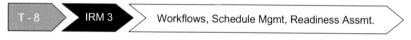

Objective

The objective of Implementation Readiness Meeting #3 (see Figure 9-14) is to continue with workflow reviews, as well as look at how schedules may be impacted at go-live. This is also a good time to assess where users stand with their level of acceptance with the technology and to surface any potential resistance to the preparation process.

Timing

Eight weeks before go-live.

Duration

Four hours in duration. Workflow discussions become intense and require much discussion among team members. Key stakeholders may be invited to the meeting, as workflow integration points may involve other departments or functions within the organization such as, but not limited to, pharmacy, lab, radiology and business services.

Details

In an ambulatory setting, because users will be working on a reduced schedule for the first weeks of go-live, it is especially helpful to invite department schedulers to this meeting to discuss what physician schedules will look like during implementation. It is important to confirm the schedules at this time, because physician schedules are typically determined two to three months in advance. With reduced schedules, it is a good idea to bring in extra staff during and post-live to help ensure patient access isn't adversely impacted. Physicians and other team members appreciate having extra staff on hand during their transition back to a full schedule.

One option is to increase hours of per diem physicians or identify interested staff physicians to work extra hours to support another facility or team go-live. In addition to helping to ensure patient care is well-supported during implementation, these physicians have the opportunity to experience an implementation before going live themselves. This is similar to the Paying It Forward suggestion described earlier and is a great way to engage early adopters in your medical group. Physicians appreciate and respond favorably to support offered by their peers, so this technique goes a long way toward accelerating the transition process for them.

During the meeting, more focus is placed on reviewing workflows and perhaps conducting relevant system demonstrations again. Although several implementation readiness meetings are slotted for workflow discussions, work outside of these meetings is required to refine the workflows. Generally workflow conferences are established with an arrangement in which team representatives are excused from the unit to work through the remaining workflow modifications, which are then reviewed during the scheduled implementation readiness meetings. Experience shows that workflows are one of the biggest problems after go-live. To avoid this, ensure your teams place enough emphasis on ensuring workflows were modified to take advantage of the new technology.

Implementation Readiness Meeting #3 is also a convenient time to assess the team's overall engagement and level of buy-in. A brief survey (as shown in Figure 9-15) is administered at this time by the ORT to gauge perceptions and uncover any potential resistance that might stand in the way of future meetings and training. Knowing what people are thinking at this point in the game is critical because you still have enough time to address any lingering negativity and/or unwillingness to participate. Encountering these issues during go-live is much too late, making it hard to intervene and get people back on track.

It is important for sponsors to continue encouraging users to take their WBT. Many users say they had to take the WBT several times before they began to feel comfortable with the system's capabilities. Sponsors themselves should take the WBT multiple times throughout the readiness process and share how this is helping in their own development. Users generally find new things that interest them every time they take the WBT, and each implementation readiness meeting will cover new topics and generate more questions about the system. Viewing the WBT multiple times can help reduce user anxiety. Of course, this process strongly relies on the user's initiative to learn about the system, unless it is mandated.

Note: This readiness assessment uses a five-point response scale. Another option is to reduce the scale to four points, eliminating the "Neutral/Undecided" option. A four-point response scale forces a favorable or unfavorable response and mitigates the risk that a respondent answers neutrally because he/she is disengaged. But for the purposes of assessing user readiness for an EMR implementation and identifying potential resistance, we prefer the five-point scale, as the "Neutral/Undecided" response is actually useful information.

Figure 9-15: Sample Readiness Assessment

SA = Strongly Agree
A = Agree
N = Neutral/Undecided
D = Disagree
SD = Strongly Disagree

#	Question	SA	A	N	D	SD
1	I understand the importance of the EMR to our organization's success.	❑	❑	❑	❑	❑
2	I know who to contact with feedback and concerns I may have about my preparation.	❑	❑	❑	❑	❑
3	I know how workflows affecting me will change.	❑	❑	❑	❑	❑
4	I can communicate the EMR benefits for patients in terms of information, quality, and safety.	❑	❑	❑	❑	❑
5	I am either comfortable with my level of PC proficiency or am preparing to improve my PC skills before go-live.	❑	❑	❑	❑	❑
6	I feel confident that I will be able to successfully learn the necessary EMR skills.	❑	❑	❑	❑	❑
7	I am encouraged and supported to attend EMR-related events and meetings.	❑	❑	❑	❑	❑
8	I take responsibility to personally learn as much as I can about the new technology.	❑	❑	❑	❑	❑
9	I know when I am scheduled to receive EMR training.	❑	❑	❑	❑	❑
10	I know what support I will receive throughout training and go-live.	❑	❑	❑	❑	❑
11	I am open to change even if it is uncomfortable at times.	❑	❑	❑	❑	❑
12	My leaders have clearly articulated the business case or rationale for why this change is needed.	❑	❑	❑	❑	❑
13	I know the changes to policies and procedures for my department.	❑	❑	❑	❑	❑
14	I know how my schedule will be affected during go-live and ramp up.	❑	❑	❑	❑	❑
15	I know when the new technology will be implemented in my department.	❑	❑	❑	❑	❑
16	I am comfortable using information technology at work.	❑	❑	❑	❑	❑
17	My leaders communicate strong ownership and personal commitment for this change.	❑	❑	❑	❑	❑
18	I know my responsibilities in terms of preparation and overall success of the upcoming implementation.	❑	❑	❑	❑	❑
19	I have attended an EMR demonstration.	❑	❑	❑	❑	❑
20	The EMR system will allow me to provide better service to patients.	❑	❑	❑	❑	❑
21	The organization does a good job of communicating about the upcoming implementation.	❑	❑	❑	❑	❑
22	My leaders behave in ways that demonstrate their support for this change.	❑	❑	❑	❑	❑

Figure 9-16: User Pre-Live Readiness Meeting #4

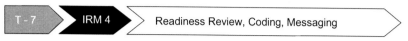

Objective

The objective of Implementation Readiness Meeting #4 (see Figure 9-16) is to review the results of the readiness assessment as a team. In addition, subject matter experts may be invited to present and/or attend the meetings to address relevant topics including, but not limited to, coding, messaging, scope of practice, and so forth.

Timing

Seven weeks before go-live.

Duration

Four hours in duration. Depending on the readiness results, the ORT and front-line leaders may need to engage in team problem solving to ensure the preparation process is meeting individual needs. There may also be various SME presentations that help connect the dots for users.

Details

Given that readiness meetings tend to be held a week apart, there is time to analyze the data from the readiness survey and review them with the team leads prior to User Pre-Live Readiness Meeting #4. The results may indicate that future meeting content needs to be modified. It is a good idea to engage the front-line supervisor in presenting the data to the team and facilitating a discussion around concerns. Users do not move progressively toward readiness when they feel their concerns are not being addressed or when they feel things are moving too quickly. Make sure you dedicate enough time for discussion in your readiness meetings. These discussions enable users to sort out their confusion and resistance in a healthy manner.

The Implementation Readiness Model lists suggested discussion topics for each meeting, but exactly when specific topics are covered may vary from organization to organization. For the fourth meeting, the model recommends deeper discussion about coding and preparing users to introduce the system to patients during go-live. You must ensure users are ready to deliver a consistent, positive elevator speech that promotes the system.

Some organizations choose to introduce specialized training in which clinicians learn how to utilize a computer when a patient is present. Without appropriate training, clinicians can alienate patients and unknowingly make them feel ignored during a visit. Using a computer in the exam room is a new concept for some people, and it is wise to orient clinicians to appropriate use to prevent the patient care experience from being compromised.

You may also want to include other stakeholder groups or SMEs in your meetings when it is useful to review handoffs and/or integration points that may be changing. The coding department, pharmacy, lab, patient safety, and other key stakeholder groups may want time on your agenda to hold these discussions. We highly recommend that you do this as it gets everyone on the same page. This is also a great way to enhance relationships, which will serve you well throughout the implementation process.

If other teams or departments have already gone live in your region, hospital, facility, or department, invite representatives from those teams to the implementation readiness meetings to discuss their experiences and how the system is impacting operations. This first-hand report provides useful information and can reduce anxiety for the team preparing to go-live. Talking with peers and colleagues about lessons learned is time well spent.

Figure 9-17: User Pre-Live Readiness Meeting #5

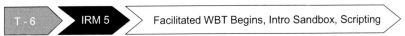

T - 6   IRM 5   Facilitated WBT Begins, Intro Sandbox, Scripting

Objective

The objective of Implementation Readiness Meeting #5 (see Figure 9-17) is to initiate preliminary training and to hold discussions around necessary scripting. This is the time that a practice environment (i.e., sandbox) is introduced to provide a safe place for users to freely navigate. Most users get a lot of value from being able touch the system, as opposed to just seeing and hearing about it.

Timing

Six weeks before go-live.

Duration

Four hours in duration. Workflow discussions continue, and facilitated WBT begins for users. This training format is very helpful for users, as they have a chance to learn at their own pace, with support. The difference between this and the WBT recommended during the first weeks is that this WBT is facilitated by support resources from the project team and operations that are there to field questions and provide help.

Details

With six weeks left before implementation, users should have viewed the WBT on their own time, reviewed the videos and participated in a facilitated WBT session. This initial training helps users acclimate to the advanced training that will be delivered closer to go-live. As a side note, detailed core systems training will be delivered throughout subsequent implementation readiness sessions, but the extensive training happens closer to go-live. Just-in-time learning has become a best practice in the industry because there is so much to learn that when training is conducted too early, users forget the skills. This is generally due to the inability to use the skills for real before go-live. Practicing skills and using them when it counts are significantly different things.

Many users say the early Web-based training really helped them retain skills learned during the advanced systems training at go-live. Having a fundamental knowledge of system capabilities is also extremely helpful for users during the readiness meetings. It enables more sophisticated questioning and better workflow decision making.

As said earlier, a common problem is that many people do not take the initiative to learn on their own. It wastes everyone else's time when unprepared users dominate classroom training with questions, keeping their colleagues from getting what they need. Additionally, these people are not value-added contributors to workflow discussions in the readiness meetings because they are uninformed about how the system works. Make sure users have taken the WBT on their own time, at least once, before participating in the facilitated WBT session.

Figure 9-18: User Pre-Live Readiness Meeting #6

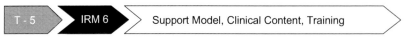

T - 5   IRM 6   Support Model, Clinical Content, Training

Objective

The objective of Implementation Readiness Meeting #6 (see Figure 9-18) is to continue with workflow reviews, as well as look at how support will be provided on the unit during the weeks of go-live. Further training is introduced to users and generally the focus centers on the importance and usefulness of establishing personalized content within the system.

Timing

Five weeks before go-live.

Duration

Four hours in duration.

Details

This meeting occurs just five weeks away from the big event. With all the discussion about workflows and the start of system-related training, users find comfort in learning how they will be supported during implementation. This is a good time to invite a representative from the support team to review support ratios and availability. Typically, support is weaned off in weeks two and three after go-live. It is extremely important that users understand this and fully engage in their preparation and readiness process. Early adopters, super users and other informal champions will be available after go-live, but the extra support will drop off at some point. It is a good idea to stress the importance of taking the readiness process seriously because users will be expected to meet performance goals shortly after they make the transition to the EMR. Make sure they are aware they must take full advantage of the support provided early on because it will not always be available to them in the same manner.

Fantastic tools are available in most EMRs to increase efficiencies and streamline processes, such as documenting in a chart or ordering procedures, medications and ancillary services. These tools operate from decision-tree logic and rely on system content. Some organizations take the time up-front to identify department-specific content, and others choose to let users customize their own content (or both). Users can take advantage of the time provided in the readiness meetings to personalize their own content, which will help at go-live *only* if they understand how to access and leverage this content.

Because the experience of go-live can be so mentally consuming to most users, their focus is truly about getting through their day. Limited attention is placed on accessing their personalized content. Our advice is to introduce the concept of personalized content in the readiness meetings, then revisit it with supplemental training a few weeks after implementation. Users approach their personalized content differently after go-live, because they have a better understanding of its advantages and application after some real experience. This increases their interest in finding more efficient ways to accomplish tasks.

Figure 9-19: User Pre-Live Readiness Meeting #7

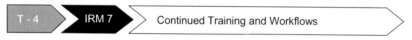

Objective

The objective of Implementation Readiness Meeting #7 (see Figure 9-19) is to continue with workflow reviews and provide more opportunity to take Web-based fundamental training.

Timing

Four weeks before go-live.

Duration

Two to four hours in duration.

Details

As stated earlier, workflows can be the biggest challenge at go-live if not properly reviewed and modified beforehand. Even if the team completes all the workflow decisions, it is a good idea to review them once more. It also helps to furnish hard copies of workflow documentation, so users can follow along, make notes as needed, and have the copies for future reference. Create a workflow binder for everyone on the team and when workflows change, replace old versions with updated versions.

Note: Most users do not have Microsoft Visio or PowerPoint on their computers, so don't rely on these only. Visual diagrams are helpful, but workflows in an outline format are useful too. With the outline format, front-line leaders can ensure the documents are easily updated when workflows need to be adjusted in the future. When users must rely on resources outside of their team to update the documents, the updates don't happen in a timely manner. It is important to keep your workflow documentation current, so everyone understands and so that new employees can be effectively oriented to the team.

Figure 9-20: User Pre-Live Readiness Meeting #8

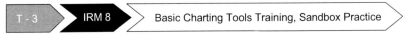

T - 3   IRM 8   Basic Charting Tools Training, Sandbox Practice

Objective

The objective of Implementation Readiness Meeting #8 (see Figure 9-20) is to ensure every user has login instructions and knows how to access and use the sandbox (the practice EMR environment that mimics the live production site). The sandbox may be open to users weeks before this readiness meeting, but it is important to provide time for users to utilize the practice environment when trainers are available to coach and guide the process. Users also begin the training cycle with instructor-led training (ILT) during week eight because go-live is around the corner. The objective is to embrace a just-in-time training approach to best accommodate the complex nature of an EMR and the myriad of new skills that need to be learned and remembered.

Timing

Three weeks before go-live.

Duration

Four hours in duration. Workflow discussions may continue and training is provided regarding charting skills and InBasket management. After training, the majority of the time should be spent on allowing users to practice in the sandbox environment. Typically, users complain of limited time to practice, so having four hours of dedicated time is very beneficial. By this time, early adopters have taken advantage of the sandbox on their own time. All users are encouraged to use the sandbox on their own time, but users frequently report that they just couldn't find the time to practice. The week eight meeting is mostly dedicated to practice, but one session is not sufficient for go-live preparation. Users must take the initiative to re-take the WBT, view the online video demonstrations, and practice as much as they can. All of this pre-work has the added advantage of preparing users to formulate sophisticated, relevant questions during their ILT sessions.

Details

Individuals can practice at their own pace in the training room or even practice as a group. It is most beneficial when they noodle through a workflow together, using the system, without direction from the facilitator. That is, the team practices its workflows as the screen is projected on the wall in front of the group. A physician or nurse drives the computer navigation, while the rest of the team members offer their thoughts on next steps. When questions surface, the facilitator can jump in and provide direction or assistance. However, it is important to stress that the facilitator should give the group the opportunity to figure out the steps on their own and not jump in to help too quickly. Enabling users to think through the processes and support themselves is a critical step in their development, and this tends to be a huge missed opportunity in some training strategies.

In an acute care environment, the luxury of attending facilitated weekly sessions may not be as easily accomplished as in an ambulatory setting. The ORT and operational leaders need to be creative and find ways for users to support one another on the unit or provide backfill to provide users with some dedicated practice time during business hours. Perhaps a rolling schedule of practice time can be established during which users have access to dedicated offices or areas at the nurses station to practice privately without interruption. Staffing the practice area with a few support resources is helpful so users can conveniently get help as questions or issues arise. Users in an inpatient setting may not be able to take a lot of time away from their work, so the idea is to try to provide them with multiple but shorter opportunities to squeeze in practice time. Sponsors play a big role in making this happen by actively dedicating computers, providing backfill, and coordinating the schedule so that support resources can be available throughout the day.

Figure 9-21: User Pre-Live Readiness Meeting #9

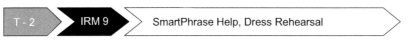

| T - 2 | IRM 9 | SmartPhrase Help, Dress Rehearsal |

Objective

The objective of Implementation Readiness Meeting #9 (see Figure 9-21) is to actually simulate a realistic scenario in which users play out their roles in the exam room, nurses' station, and/or physician office by following department-specific and role-specific workflows.

Timing

Two weeks before go-live.

Duration

Four hours in duration. Do not provide less than four hours to conduct the dress rehearsal. The more time devoted to this preparation technique, the better.

Details

By now, users have had multiple opportunities to learn about the system, have taken the WBT on their own time, attended a facilitated WBT session, viewed online video demonstrations, worked with their respective teams to confirm new workflows, attended live workflow demonstrations, received basic system training, and have practiced these newfound skills and workflows in the system. Although they will receive deeper systems training closer to go-live, at this point users should already have a good foundational set of skills with the system and workflows and be ready to take their preparation to the next level.

The dress rehearsal is a critical element in any implementation readiness program, but it is frequently overlooked because of the time and effort involved in planning and arranging it. Nonetheless, users are far more effective using the new technology when they have had ample opportunities to practice in scenarios that closely match real-life conditions.

Think about a dress rehearsal during a wedding. The wedding party conducts a dry run of the ceremony. The wedding facilitator helps everyone involved understand their role, where to stand, and what to do during the ceremony. This is similar to a technology implementation dress rehearsal, and users benefit greatly from dry runs of workflows and scenarios that frequently occur in their daily operations. The learning is most relevant and sustainable when the dress rehearsal is conducted on the team's own unit. Do not conduct it anywhere else.

In an acute care setting, it is more challenging to conduct the dress rehearsal than in the ambulatory setting. In acute care the dress rehearsal is sometimes done on the floor in a dedicated area, but there will likely be real patients surrounding these dedicated practice sites. Although the acute care dress rehearsal is logistically more challenging, it actually has the benefit of more closely mimicking a real-life scenario. Our recommendation is to maintain flexibility through the dress rehearsal process. You may be faced with interruptions and might even need to postpone completing the dress rehearsal if a patient situation arises and colleagues need help. Patient safety and care always come first! (See page 172 for one organization's approach to inpatient dress rehearsal.)

The ORT works closely with operational leaders and the implementation project team to develop department-specific scripts that will guide the dress rehearsal. The scripts should outline a typical day-in-the-life of the user, from patient intake to patient discharge. In an ambulatory setting three people should be assigned to an exam room—a physician, a nurse, and a patient. The script provides everything that should be said by the participating individuals, including how patients are greeted and roomed in real life. The facilitator and/or trainer may play one of the three roles or choose to be an onlooker.

As in an earlier Implementation Readiness Meeting, the facilitator and/or trainer must not intervene too often but rather step in if confusion or questions arise. Users must work together to fulfill their roles in the dress rehearsal, making decisions that they will use in real life.

Again, the objective is to enable the users to think through the process and try to solve their own problems before having real patients in the mix. A common preparation pitfall is for facilitators and trainers to intervene too regularly. Although well-intended, the impact is actually counterproductive because it impedes the critical thinking and learning process that must take place for users.

Successful practice ideas:

- Have doctors and nurses switch roles during dress rehearsal to experience each others' process. This is a valuable and revealing learning experience.
- Dress rehearsal is a good opportunity for the facilitator/trainer to identify those having problems completing the test scenarios and arrange to give them extra help before go-live.

Figure 9-22: User Pre-Live Readiness Meeting #10

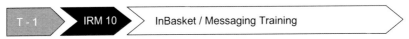

T - 1   IRM 10   InBasket / Messaging Training

Objective

The objective of Implementation Readiness Meeting #10 (see Figure 9-22) is to begin advanced system training. Training is best retained when conducted close to go-live.

Timing

One week before go-live.

Duration

Four hours in duration, allowing ample time for questions and discussions.

Details

At this point, users should have a solid understanding of what the organization is envisioning and how they fit into the bigger picture. Also, the context for learning should be well-supported, with front-line supervisors reinforcing desired behaviors and performance expectations. It is most effective when front-line supervisors are present during the core training sessions to field any outstanding issues or work-flow questions.

Advanced training exists beyond go-live and continues through-out the first, and in some cases, the second week of going live. Users work to assimilate everything they have learned and make informed decisions regarding the best ways to utilize the system to fulfill organizational expectations and meet the needs of their patients.

3. GO-LIVE TEAM TRAINING

Figure 9-23: Stage Three of the Implementation Readiness Program

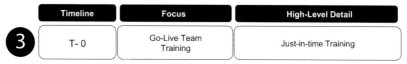

As highlighted in Figure 9-23, the focus of the third stage of the Implementation Readiness Program is to provide just-in-time training.

Figure 9-24: Go-live!

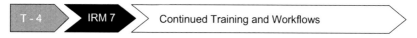

Objective

An Implementation Readiness Meeting (see Figure 9-24) is held the day of go-live because the preparation process continues. Users receive advanced, comprehensive training the morning of go-live and then go back to their floor or unit to work a reduced schedule or workload. A team debrief is scheduled at the close of the shift.

Timing

Day of go-live.

Duration

Four hours training in the morning, reduced schedule or workload, one hour debrief meeting at the end of the shift.

Details

This is it! Go-live has arrived. Users receive advanced system training in the morning and reduced schedules or workload in the afternoon. The training reinforces earlier training, but it also addresses any logon issues and other questions the team may have before using the EMR for the first time with real patients. During the training, it is important to remind users that support resources are nearby to support them through the day. The difference between the training received at go-live and prior training sessions is that the Systems Training #1 focuses on bringing all of the training together. Users are asked to work through pre-scripted scenarios that are relevant to their role and specialty. In a sense, it is training and practice all wrapped into one with the intent to build user confidence that they can do it!

Executive sponsors play a huge role at go-live and should be present at the go-live training, as well as being visible during go-live on the unit or floor. Users appreciate the moral support. It also reinforces how important this implementation is, so important that the senior executives are on hand to show their appreciation for all of the hard work of preparing for this transition.

Team debriefs are critical at the end of the day of go-live and during subsequent readiness efforts. This enables users to unwind and share their experiences, frustrations, and thoughts about the go-live experience. This forum must be provided so users are not left to their own devices to sort out what just happened to them. Also, it is important to surface any potential issues or outstanding levels of resistance, so the sponsors, front-line supervisors, and support team can intervene effectively. Team debriefs are helpful for users to reach closure for the day and gives them renewed energy for tomorrow.

4. POST-LIVE TEAM MEETINGS

The day of go-live is just the beginning to the overall transition and change that users will experience (see Figure 9-25). The act of installing the system is not the final stage of implementation. Many argue

Figure 9-25: Stage Four of Implementation Readiness Program

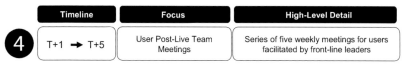

Timeline	Focus	High-Level Detail
4 T+1 ➡ T+5	User Post-Live Team Meetings	Series of five weekly meetings for users facilitated by front-line leaders

that life actually begins after go-live. As such, the preparation continues with five more weeks of recommended training and team debriefs, as shown in Figure 9-26.

The post-implementation focus is on more advanced system training and ensuring team debriefs are occurring on a regular basis. Users are now applying their newfound skills and knowledge in a real-life setting, and they are becoming more sophisticated in their utilization of the technology. New questions are coming up, along with ideas for improvement. This is not the time to reduce support. Users need to stabilize and increase their level of confidence. And those who are struggling must not be allowed to fall further behind. Holding forums during which teams speak openly about their experiences and collaborate on solutions is a valuable part of the preparation process and also help teams begin to support themselves.

The five post-implementation meetings will not be reviewed individually because the purpose of these meetings is the same: bring the team together in a supportive environment, provide opportunity for open discussion and problem solving, and deliver additional training. Support resources should be focused on working with front-line leaders to ensure they are comfortable in their roles and that they have the

Figure 9-26: Post-Implementation Preparation Model

T + 1	PIM 1	System Training #2, Team Debrief #2
T + 2	PIM 2	Advanced Charting Skills, Team Debrief #3
T + 3	PIM 3	Supplemental Training, Team Debrief #4
T + 4	PIM 4	Team Debrief #5
T + 5	PIM 5	Follow Up InBasket / Messaging Training

tools and resources to manage team performance. Strong leaders have strong teams, so effort to coach and mentor front-line leaders, as well as their teams, must continue.

The Implementation Readiness Model is based on a significant amount of experience implementing software implementations, but it is important to note that it is not a cookie-cutter approach. That is, every organization is different and should customize the model to account for the culture, business priorities, actual software/applications to be implemented, and other operational considerations. It is great to see the latest developments, innovations, and creative solutions that organizations are generating to effectively prepare users for an EMR implementation. Some rather successful practices are in place and are still emerging. Consider the following two successful practices.

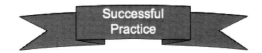

NorthShore University HealthSystem's Approach to Training for Their EMR Implementation

NorthShore has a Chief Learning Officer who is part of Human Resources, and that person led the EMR training effort and spent a lot of time teaching clinicians how to teach adults.

We made training mandatory for all levels of employees and medical staff. Our professional staff passed a rule that said you need to use Epic to take care of patients in the hospital and that you can't use Epic without passing the course. That applied to our employed physicians, as well as to community physicians who admit patients to our facilities.

We offered basic computer training for anyone who was uncomfortable with a mouse, etc. We did this privately, and I am sure many went to their kids for help as well. We didn't want to embarrass them in the class, and we didn't want them slowing down the class.

Go-live Training

Things changed over time, but for the first three hospitals that came up on the EMR, we required in-classroom training. We offered two options—

either four-hour classes over four consecutive days or eight-hour classes over two days, with both days occurring on the weekend. Overall, the idea was that if we were going to disrupt their day, we should at least let them pick the time.

The exam was competency-based; they had to demonstrate that they knew what to do. Physicians took the test as part of their class; we thought it would be hard to get them back one more time. Other staff returned to their departments and were given access to a practice environment. We then asked their super user to do the competency exams. We wanted the departments to tell us that their staff was ready, not us telling them.

We did almost all of this training off-site, so it was impossible to lose a doctor to answering a page and going to the floor. We also offered refresher training, since it was impossible to train everyone close enough to go-live.

Our departmental chairmen and their opinion leaders attended the first session, and they all passed. It was hard after that for any other doctors to say that they didn't have the time or could not pass the test.

We used floaters in the classrooms. These were people who were not teaching but checking on students to be sure they were on the right screens and offering quiet help to be sure students could move along and keep up. Some of these floaters were physicians who were our physician advisory committee members. For the current go-live, we have recruited and given extra training to some of their opinion leaders to perform this floating role.

Training Now

Online training is now available for physicians in our original three hospitals. We needed to do this to allow rotating house staff to be ready when they came on site. Many of the house staff have had access to Epic or other EMRs at other hospitals. They were joining a group of users on a floor or in a department who were already experienced users of Epic (herd immunity).

A new hospital is joining us in December that has no herd immunity, so we've returned to classroom training for these physicians.

Upgrades/New Releases

The amount of training for any new functionality factors into our decision on what we bring live each year. We need to be sure that we can train the staff on the new functionality or module. This is often the limiting factor in what we include in an upgrade.

The training needs and team are part of our work plan discussions and not an afterthought. We now have hospital-based trainers who come to your elbow after being paged. They do not have classroom responsibility. Some of our users take advantage of this service to learn a newer, more advanced feature. Others who do not come to the hospitals often and don't have Epic in their office, use it to get through an admission.

Tom Smith
CIO
NorthShore University HealthSystem
Evanston, Illinois

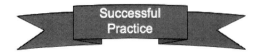

BayCare Health System's Approach to Training for Their EMR Implementation

It is extremely important to align all activities that focus on the "people-side" of EMR implementation early in project planning. All activities necessary for ultimate adoption of system and cultural change must be planned and intentional. They must build on the successful completion of prior tasks, allowing team members and leadership to clearly envision each stepping stone on the path to transformation.

One activity that has proven successful within an inpatient setting is the utilization of a "mock practice" or "dress rehearsal" prior to activation of the new workflow processes and technology. This activity entails using real patient data documented in a non-production environment running parallel to the delivery of clinical care within the patient's room or appropriate clinical area. In other words, a nurse, accompanied by someone from the support team, delivers patient care and uses a practice site in the process to approximate what will happen at go-live and thereafter. Care must be taken to ensure that each team member participating in the rehearsal has completed all training requirements and clearly understands all objectives and requirements to completing the rehearsal. Patients and other providers were made aware that a "practice" session was being completed within their area. Signs were posted stating "Experienced Nurse, New Computer System" to help patients and visitors understand that the new system was being implemented. There are many factors that come into play when planning this type of activity, and alignment of key project and facility/user personnel is elemental to success.

Once the decision to incorporate this type of activity into your activation has been solidified, the work can begin. Stakeholders will come to the table eager to see every piece of functionality, from every part of the system, in every workflow scenario possible, and in every impacted area. The first step of this planning is to help "scope" what is both appropriate for the size and magnitude of the implementation and what is feasible from a preparation and support model. We have found it very successful to be open to suggestions and recommendations but finalize all agreed activities within a brief scope document. This helps align expectations across all parties. The key to success is to have all parties clearly understand the logistics, preparation, and expected outcome of the rehearsal.

A few key factors to help guide your team in scope decisions might include:

- *What are other activities that are going on within the facility (e.g., training, device deployment, other competing facility initiatives)?*
- *When should this rehearsal begin (date and time of day)?*
- *Which departments will be included in the rehearsal, which depends greatly on the overall scope of your activation (e.g., ED, Radiology, Lab, Telemetry, Pharmacy…)?*
- *How many participants will be involved (nurses, physicians, techs, etc.)?*
- *How many visitors will you allow to observe the activity without disrupting patient flow/satisfaction (many others will want to see the system)?*
- *How long will the activity run (12, 24, 36, or 48 hours)?*

- *How will the project team provide support to the facility during the rehearsal (e.g., at-the-elbow support, remote production/security support)?*
- *Will there be extra staff brought in to provide patient care, while those involved in the activity are allowed to "practice" real-life scenarios within the practice domain of your system (how many, who pays their time, skill sets needed)?*

A few key objectives to this type of activity that help obtain buy-in from all parties include:

- *Validating the future state design to meet end-user operational needs.*
- *Obtaining end-user input on how the system will work in their daily working environment.*
- *Pre-testing the activation support procedures and model.*
- *Providing the best, and most thorough, opportunity to validate overall flow of data, availability of data for viewing, and hardware usage.*

A few key benefits that come out of dress rehearsals include:

- *End-users will use the system in a real patient care setting and identify issues or gaps that need mitigation prior to go-live.*
- *Provides "practical practice" for end-users post-training.*
- *Provides an opportunity for go-live support to have practical experience with their support role.*
- *End-users become familiar with new devices/device functionality.*
- *End-users can use this opportunity to practice what they have learned. This helps highlight those areas of training that need additional emphasis or job aides.*
- *Validation of production support and device strategies occurs.*
- *Informal wireless devices are tested.*
- *Solidifies "buy-in" from facility/department leadership.*

Ronnie D. Bower, Jr., MA
Manager, Change Management
BayCare Health System

Section IV

Summary

CHAPTER 10

The Journey

You can't make an omelet without breaking any eggs.

An EMR implementation can take on a life of its own, so it is extremely important to understand what you are getting into and prepare well for the journey. The lessons shared in this book are based on years of experience managing the people side of many software deployment projects (not to mention the largest private healthcare organization EMR implementation in the world!). The intent is to help you plan and experience a meaningful implementation and achieve new heights for your organization. The quality of your journey will be determined by how well you establish a supportive context for change and manage the people side of the implementation.

We conclude this book with a final set of thoughts and recommendations and wish you a smooth journey to EMR benefit realization.

OWNERSHIP

One of the hardest things for any organization embarking on an EMR implementation is to understand that an implementation of this sort is a business initiative, not an IT project. This is an extremely important concept because, as we have said repeatedly in this book, the EMR itself isn't what is important. The critical factor is whether the technology is embraced and used once it is installed. It's counterproductive for organizations to place so much emphasis on installing the technology that they don't take the time to make sure it is fully adopted and incorporated into daily operations. To avoid this problem, create a strong partnership between IT and operations, with operations as the owner and IT as the enabler.

If strong and active engagement from operations and senior leadership is not present, escalate the issue to the project steering committee. You may need to reassess the effectiveness of executive sponsorship or even re-evaluate the level of engagement from the steering committee. If operations doesn't take ownership of the EMR, the journey through implementation and beyond will be long, arduous, and frustrating, and you run a significant risk that the initiative will fail.

MANAGING PERCEPTIONS

The EMR system presents tremendous transformative potential for an organization. But, if users feel the technology is "being forced down their throats," or if they aren't sold on the value proposition, it will be difficult to generate the required level of buy-in from operations leaders and staff. Instead, a resistance will develop, and it will come from all angles. Establish an environment of open communication about the anticipated journey to get the resistance out in the open, so it can be dealt with effectively.

There are two good ways to establish an atmosphere of trust and open communication. First of all, honesty still remains the best policy, so tell people the truth about what to expect and, if you are uncertain about something, don't be afraid to say so. Users respect leaders when they tell the truth. People want to hear the real story, including anticipated benefits, risks, and potential difficulties.

Secondly, provide forums in which users feel safe sharing their thoughts, concerns, and questions. These can be team meetings, department meetings, special sessions called by the project leader, feedback loops, etc. When people have the opportunity to work out their uncertainty and issues openly, they get the information they need. This limits what they are able to "make up" and short-circuits the effectiveness of rumors. Anxious people who lack information fill the gap with speculation and half-truths. After time, these stories become believable and have the power to negatively influence the way users view and utilize the EMR. Avoid this common scenario by ensuring that users have opportunities to freely and comfortably make sense of things in a supportive environment.

POINTING FINGERS

When users resist the implementation of a new EMR, they often project their frustration and fear onto the technology and claim the EMR is the source of all of their problems.

"If only we could go back to the way things were."

The new technology creates transparency that surfaces broken processes that existed long before implementation. People are not always happy when they realize that the EMR serves as a huge magnifying glass that calls attention to problems and inefficiencies that were hidden before.

The good news is that, properly implemented and adopted, the EMR will help streamline and improve efficiency. The hard part is that people don't always want to change established processes, especially when there is some personal benefit in how things have always been done. Inevitably, the EMR becomes the object of resentment and is blamed for all the users' headaches. It is common to hear new users claim life was better before the technology.

We suggest three things. One, sometimes you have to remind people that life wasn't all that great in the past. Pick the time to say this carefully. Two, in all of our experience, we have yet to encounter anyone who gets through a few weeks post-live and wants to go back to paper or an outdated system. It just doesn't happen.

And three, we strongly recommend that *before go-live*, you make as many nonsystem related changes as possible. Do not burden the go-live process by encumbering users with changes that do not require use of the system and cause resistance.

Here's an example. In acute care settings, if one objective is to have nurses begin documenting at the bedside using the EMR, there is no reason why you can't begin bedside documentation months in advance of go-live, using the paper chart or whatever is the current method. This has several benefits. One, bedside documentation will not be blamed on the system. Two, the bugs in establishing bedside documentation practice will get worked out before go-live. And three, nurses won't have to try to use an unfamiliar system and change their documentation patterns all at the same time during go-live. The point is to make go-live as easy as possible for users, not to complicate it unnecessarily.

Identify and implement everything that can be done ahead of go-live. You and your users will be glad you did!

MANAGING AMBIGUITY

EMR implementations are full of uncertainty and ambiguity, which affects people in different ways. Some users are fine sifting through uncertain times, and others find the lack of order and answers to be very uncomfortable.

Be mindful of ambiguity and how people deal with it. Ambiguity can be very scary for users. It's a natural reaction but can spiral out of control if not managed well. You don't get the best from people when they are distracted by worry about their future. Ambiguity will always be present when things are in flux and subject to change. Manage user expectations by letting them know there will be uncertainty and what the organization is doing to find solutions to open questions; communicating honestly and frequently; soliciting and responding to feedback and getting users involved in the project.

LIFE AFTER GO-LIVE

Here's a news flash for many people—the journey never ends! In fact, things really get rolling after go-live. Don't be fooled into thinking that go-live is the big event, and life calms down afterwards. Instead, the journey continues and, depending on how well users were prepared for implementation, you may be in store for a whole lot more than you bargained for. But if a good context for change was established before go-live, the transition to post-live will be much smoother. Remember, the context is important because it creates an environment in which users are engaged and look forward to improving their skills post-implementation.

Go-live is like a wedding. Two people spend a great deal of time preparing for the big event and then look at each other when it's over and wonder where the time went (despite the many decisions and stress involved in planning the effort). The married couple now begins to settle down and learns to co-exist. With merging lifestyles and healthy sacrifices, the couple engages in life collaboratively, with both parties eager to make adjustments along the way to ensure a happy life together. The wedding is a big event but, like an EMR implementation, it's what happens afterward that really matters.

Unfortunately many optimization efforts fail to bring home anticipated returns, largely because optimization begins before users are ready for additional changes. After go-live, users need to adjust to using the system in real time with real patients. Some struggle to adapt to the new routine. Others may be stuck at go-live, trying to understand how to see a patient and use a computer at the same time. This can be a difficult period for users, and they need time and support to sort things out and stabilize. Allow them to adjust before launching enhancements and additional technology. They won't be able to grasp new skills and information when they are still trying to get comfortable with what they learned for go-live.

Life after go-live is where the action is. The organization needs to put its energy into ensuring that users are comfortable in their roles, able to use the system efficiently, and can learn how to leverage the system to contribute to outcomes. This requires a post-live strategy (and budget!) to make sure performance targets are set, expectations are communicated, outcomes are measured, and customized training and support are delivered to those who require extra help.

EMR IMPLEMENTATION RISK FACTORS

- Failure to cascade sponsorship through the organization to front-line operations.
- Not establishing a comprehensive governance structure (beyond executive sponsors) for making decisions, prioritizing, and managing the roll-out.
- Not getting medical staff, labor unions, and other key stakeholders engaged up front.
- Assigning change management/technology adoption responsibilities to technical or project management staff.
- Rewarding behavior that is inconsistent with the vision by neglecting to realign incentive programs to reinforce people for future state behaviors and outcomes.
- Not addressing the need to facilitate behavioral change by supporting people to develop new skills and new ways of thinking, in addition to learning features and functions of the software.

- Underestimating the degree of resistance that will be experienced and not preparing for it.
- Not holding sponsors accountable for effective sponsorship. Allowing sponsors to get away with not supporting the transformation.
- Thinking that technically skilled people make good champions, or selecting local champions based on title or availability instead of informal leadership ability.
- Letting past success and strengths get in the way of what needs to be done to succeed in the future. Past success may be the greatest threat to transformation.
- Letting intellectual capital (the content in consultants' or vendor implementation people's heads) walk out the door without doing comprehensive knowledge transfer. If you're getting outside help, make sure you retain as much knowledge as possible when they leave.

FINAL THOUGHTS

- Doctors and nurses communicate with each other less in the beginning stages of an implementation. They are so focused on the new EMR that they forget to talk to each other. But the EMR shouldn't be seen as a replacement for collaboration and human interaction. Counsel people about this during team readiness meetings prior to the EMR launch to avoid development of bad habits.
- It takes time for many users to overcome concern that the EMR will do their jobs for them. It is very important to reinforce that the EMR is merely a tool that will support them in their work.
- Some organizations form cross-functional workgroups to resolve important issues, instead of having leaders making all the decisions. Workgroups are a way to get others involved. Include some who are resistant to ensure all voices are heard. Members of the workgroup represent their teams and bring local input to the problem. This extends the reach of the workgroup, often resulting in broader buy-in for proposed recommendations.
- User confidence in the organization is eroded when leaders are perceived as clueless about what lies ahead and how it impacts users and departments. Knowledgeable, effective leadership reas-

sures users that all of their hard work and change will eventually lead to positive outcomes. Sponsors at all levels play an enormous role in communicating the importance of the EMR and modeling the path to a positive future state.

- One of our primary goals in writing this book is to help people see that an EMR implementation can transform the organization by building change capability and capacity. When the next big change project comes up (and it will be soon!), imagine a world in which users expect change management support, sponsors *willingly resource* the people side, and the organization has broad skills to do change management well.

- An EMR implementation is not an event; it is a long-term process which, if sustainable, never ends because the EMR becomes part of operations and is the "way we do things around here." This is another way of saying that go-live is just the beginning of the future state, not the end goal.

- Accepting the computer and openly engaging in process improvement can be threatening to people. Some organizations implement job security programs or offer a retention bonus to encourage people to look openly at opportunities for performance improvement using the EMR without feeling they are putting their jobs at risk.

- Remember to think through any potential impact to patients (such as longer wait times), particularly during go-live. People are often supportive and understanding when they know something big is going on, but you have to tell them about it. Having signage and staff on hand to answer questions and troubleshoot goes a long way in gaining patient acceptance.

- Leverage what you're got! People are busy and schedules are tight. In every way that you can, leverage existing meetings, roles, committees, task forces, and events to support the EMR effort. Avoid setting up parallel structures whenever possible.

- To the extent possible eliminate distractions before, during, and just after go-live. Successful practices include putting other projects on temporary hold, reducing e-mail volume, and canceling all non-EMR related meetings. Focus the organization's energy on the EMR deployment.

- If computers in clinical areas are a new thing in your organization, support your staff by providing them with training on effective and respectful use of the computer with a patient present.
- With EMR implementations, the idea is to find a way to ensure everyone has skin in the game regarding the success of the implementation. The skin in the game must outlive the event of go-live and carry forward through life post-live if sustainability and benefit realization are to be achieved.

We hope you have enjoyed taking this journey with us and that we have provided ideas and insights that will help you support your users and your organization through a successful electronic medical record implementation. We will continue the journey in our next book where we will address post-live optimization and benefit realization. We hope you will join us.

We welcome your comments and questions. We can be reached as follows:

Claire McCarthy
Cem820@yahoo.com

Doug Eastman
DougEastman@att.net

References

1. Bridges W. *Managing Transitions, Making the Most of Change.* Reading, MA: Addison-Wesley, 1991.

2. Kubler-Ross E. *On Death and Dying.* New York: The Macmillan Company, 1969.

3. IMA. *Accelerating Implementation Methodology (AIM);* 2009. http:www.imaworldwide.com. Accessed November 15, 2009.

4. Gostick A, Elton C. *The Carrot Principle.* New York: Free Press, 2009.

Index